AGRICULTURE ISSUES AND POLICIES

LIVE ANIMAL IMPORTS AND DISEASE

REGULATORY PRACTICES AND RECOMMENDATIONS

AGRICULTURE ISSUES AND POLICIES

Additional books in this series can be found on Nova's website under the Series tab.

Additional E-books in this series can be found on Nova's website under the E-book tab.

AGRICULTURE ISSUES AND POLICIES

LIVE ANIMAL IMPORTS AND DISEASE

REGULATORY PRACTICES AND RECOMMENDATIONS

MATT C. GRAYSON
AND
PETE A. MCLAIN
EDITORS

nova publishers
New York

For permission to use material from this book please contact us:
Telephone 631-231-7269; Fax 631-231-8175
Web Site: http://www.novapublishers.com

Library of Congress Cataloging-in-Publication Data

ISBN: 978-1-62618-275-2

Published by Nova Science Publishers, Inc. † New York

CONTENTS

PREFACE

The United States is the world's leading import market for live animals. From 2005 through 2008 more than 1 billion live animals were legally imported into the United States for agriculture, clinical research, education and exhibition, the aquarium and pet industries, and other uses. These imports have the potential to transmit zoonotic diseases; which are infectious diseases that can be transmitted between animals and humans and can cause a substantial number of deaths. The spread of zoonotic diseases, as well as other diseases affecting only animals, can take a major economic toll on many industries. This book examines potential gaps in the statutory and regulatory framework governing live animal imports, that may allow the introduction and spread of zoonotic and animal diseases, the extent to which the various government oversight agencies collaborate to meet their responsibilities on this issue, and performance information that the responsible agencies have reported on live animal imports.

Chapter 1 - The United States legally imported more than 1 billion live animals from 2005 through 2008. With increased trade and travel, zoonotic diseases (transmitted between animals and humans) and animal diseases can emerge anywhere and spread rapidly.

The importation of live animals is governed by five principal statutes and implemented by four agencies.

GAO was asked to examine, among other things, (1) potential gaps in the statutory and regulatory framework governing live animal imports, if any, that may allow the introduction and spread of zoonotic and animal diseases and (2) the extent to which the agencies collaborate to meet their responsibilities, and face barriers, if any, to collaboration.

GAO reviewed statutes, met with agency officials, visited ports of entry, and surveyed experts on animal imports.

Chapter 2 - To protect the health and welfare of our nation's animals, the U.S. Department of Agriculture's (USDA) Animal and Plant Health Inspection Service (APHIS) regulates the importation and quarantine of live animals. In fiscal year (FY) 2008, APHIS required that 165,000 high-risk animals, such as birds from countries affected by Exotic Newcastle Disease, be quarantined at either an APHIS animal import center or a private quarantine facility to ensure that they were not carrying diseases that might spread to the domestic animal population. The authors initiated this audit to evaluate APHIS' controls over the quarantine and tracking of animals at quarantine facilities, as well as the user fees APHIS charged importers to fund its facilities.

Overall, the authors concluded that APHIS needs to take steps to improve its controls over the animal import process, especially as it relates to quarantining animals that may be carrying infectious diseases. APHIS established import policies and procedures for import center officials and port staff to follow, while area officials were responsible for providing supervisory oversight of both import center and port operations. APHIS port (i.e., airport) staff monitors the arrival and transport of imported animals to a quarantine facility, where import center officials observe and test those animals for foreign diseases. APHIS import center officials also provide oversight of APHIS-approved private quarantine facilities.

The authors identified weaknesses in the procedures APHIS used to handle animals destined for a quarantine facility, beginning with the precautions it took when receiving the animals into the country and continuing to the bio-security conditions at the quarantine facilities themselves. APHIS officials did not identify these weaknesses because they did not exercise sufficient oversight to ensure import and quarantine requirements were met. Instead, they relied on the experience and expertise of port staff and import center officials. The weaknesses the authors identified significantly increased the risk that infected animals could enter the country undetected through quarantine facilities. In two instances, the authors found that birds infected with Exotic Newcastle Disease and at least one horse infected with Contagious Equine Metritis had entered the country and spread the diseases to other animals.

When animals are imported into the country, they are met by APHIS import center or port staff who review the importers' permits and health certificates. These documents are APHIS' key internal controls for identifying animals that should be placed into a quarantine facility for observation and determining whether certain precautions should be taken. The authors found problems with these controls for 53 of 131 shipments selected for review. APHIS import center and port staff did not (1) follow permit instructions which required the shipments to be monitored while they were being transferred from ports-of-entry to the quarantine facility, (2) ensure that health certificates included all required information about the animals, or (3) record the correct country of origin on the permit application for some shipments.

APHIS area officials had not performed periodic reviews of port operations. Area officials trusted port staff to ensure compliance with prescribed agency procedures related to the import of animals, including imports from countries that require additional certification, handling, testing, or quarantine. APHIS established these requirements to reduce the risk that animals imported from countries affected by disease would infect our nation's domestic animal population. Thus, it is crucial that port staff adheres to these requirements to prevent the unnecessary importation and subsequent spread of a foreign animal disease. For instance, one of the shipments in the authors' review included birds infected with Exotic Newcastle Disease, which is a highly contagious viral disease that is 100 percent fatal to all species of birds. When those birds came into contact with other birds in quarantine, APHIS had to euthanize more than 9,000 birds.

APHIS port staff had also not always followed the agency's regulations concerning proper sanitation at ports-of-entry. These sanitation procedures included monitoring the cleaning and disinfecting cargo areas and equipment, and collecting debris that may harbor a foreign animal disease. APHIS area officials relied on the port staff's experience and expertise and, therefore, did not periodically review the port's sanitation procedures. At three of the four airports the authors visited, APHIS port staff did not follow proper sanitation procedures since they did not ensure that aircraft cargo areas and transport equipment were cleaned and disinfected, and non-APHIS personnel were wearing protective clothing. The authors observed individuals in shorts and sandals handling foreign animals bound for quarantine facilities. Proper sanitation procedures are important to prevent the spread of foreign animal disease beyond the port-of-entry or from physically affecting the individuals handling these animals.

The APHIS animal import centers and agency-approved private quarantine facilities the authors visited had physical security deficiencies that increased the risk of spreading a foreign animal disease outside the facility. These deficiencies included single-entry rather than self-closing double doors; torn or inadequate screens over windows and doors; individuals who were not showering as they entered and exited facilities; and contractors that were not disinfecting vehicles when they exited facilities. In addition, five of the six private facilities the authors visited were not adequately accounting for birds brought into quarantine.

The authors found that APHIS had not developed bio-security procedures for its animal import centers to follow because it relied on the experience and expertise of import center officials to use good judgment. In addition, even though APHIS had written bio-security requirements for private quarantine facilities, it did not identify or require those facilities to correct quarantine violations. The authors attributed the deficiencies at private quarantine facilities to agency import center officials who, even though they were aware of the violations, did not enforce agency policies. APHIS officials did not correct the import center officials' actions because they did not review import center operations or the centers' oversight of private quarantine facilities. APHIS officials stated that the quarantine deficiencies the authors noted should have been corrected.

Further, APHIS area officials were not aware of deficiencies at either type of quarantine facility because APHIS did not require them to review, and had not itself reviewed, animal import center operations or their oversight of private quarantine facilities since 2005.

APHIS area officials were not directly overseeing private quarantine facilities for horses that were being imported from countries affected by Contagious Equine Metritis. APHIS had not required its area officials to oversee those facilities because it relied on State agencies to approve and monitor facilities that quarantine horses.

In 2007, APHIS officials performed an internal review that noted this lack of oversight and recommended that agency officials review and monitor State activities. In 2009, APHIS officials acknowledged that an imported horse with the disease passed through one of these State-approved private facilities. That horse infected 27 domestic horses and exposed almost 1,000 more to the disease.

Finally, the authors questioned the methodology APHIS used to calculate the fees it charged importers for agency quarantine services. The agency's current methodology for determining its user fee rates was insufficient to cover operating costs and provide for capital improvements that facilities need to meet basic bio-security requirements.

APHIS had established the user fee rate based on a 1995 time study, which is no longer accurate because it significantly understates the time it takes for agency employees to perform quarantine tasks. According to an

APHIS official, the time aspect of the user fee rate had not been updated because it was assumed that the tasks and the time to complete them had not changed since 1995.

The inadequate methodology contributed, in part, to the agency's budget shortfall because operating expenses at animal import centers exceeded revenues by $1.6 million from FY's 2004 through 2008. The animal import centers also had deferred many maintenance and capital improvement projects that jeopardized the physical security of the quarantine facilities.

Overall, the authors concluded that APHIS needs to improve its oversight of the animal import process to ensure compliance with prescribed agency procedures, especially with respect to animals from countries that require additional certification, handling, testing, or quarantine.

In addition, APHIS needs to periodically review and amend its user fee structure to ensure animal import centers have the financial ability to complete maintenance and capital improvement projects related to the physical security of quarantine facilities.

Chapter 3 - Internet commerce (hereafter e-commerce) is a growing and vital part of the U.S. economy. Total e-commerce sales in the U.S. for 2011 totaled $194 billion, an increase of 16% over 2010. From 2002 to 2011, the proportion of reported e-commerce sales in the U.S. grew from about 1.4% to 5.5% of total retail sales (U.S. Census Bureau News 2012). Globally, e-commerce is expected to increase at a rate of 13.5% annually, amounting to $1.4 trillion in yearly sales by 2015 (Enright 2011). A portion of this activity includes the sale and trade of living organisms. Unfortunately, such organisms and other organisms that they may carry can be invasive species, defined by U.S. Executive Order 131121 as "alien [non-native] species whose introduction does or is likely to cause economic or environmental harm or harm to human health." Order 131121 mandates that Federal agencies work to ensure that they do not promote e-commerce in invasive species, because the order states that these agencies should..."not authorize, fund, or carry out actions that are likely to cause or promote the introduction or spread of invasive species...."

A number of government entities have jurisdiction over aspects of e-commerce including particular types of organisms (U.S. Department of Agriculture, Animal and Plant Health Inspection Service [USDA, APHIS] – plants, livestock and their products; Department of Interior [DOI], U.S. Fish and Wildlife Service [USFWS] – wildlife); shipping services (Department of Homeland Security [DHS], U.S. Postal Service [USPS]); imports and interstate trade (Federal government) and intrastate trade (state governments). However, e-commerce as a sector is evolving and expanding in volume at a rate that may exceed these various capacities to address the associated risks of introduction and spread of invasive species.

In: Live Animal Imports and Disease
Editors: M. Grayson and P. McLain
ISBN: 978-1-62618-275-2

Chapter 1

LIVE ANIMAL IMPORTS: AGENCIES NEED BETTER COLLABORATION TO REDUCE THE RISK OF ANIMAL-RELATED DISEASES*

United States Government Accountability Office

WHY GAO DID THIS STUDY

The United States legally imported more than 1 billion live animals from 2005 through 2008. With increased trade and travel, zoonotic diseases (transmitted between animals and humans) and animal diseases can emerge anywhere and spread rapidly.

The importation of live animals is governed by five principal statutes and implemented by four agencies.

GAO was asked to examine, among other things, (1) potential gaps in the statutory and regulatory framework governing live animal imports, if any, that may allow the introduction and spread of zoonotic and animal diseases and (2) the extent to which the agencies collaborate to meet their responsibilities, and face barriers, if any, to collaboration.

GAO reviewed statutes, met with agency officials, visited ports of entry, and surveyed experts on animal imports.

---

* This is an edited, reformatted and augmented version of United States Government Accountability Office, Publication No. GAO-11-9, dated November 2010.

What GAO Recommends

GAO recommends that the Secretaries of Agriculture, Health and Human Services, Homeland Security, and the Interior develop a strategy to address barriers to agency collaboration that may allow potentially risky imported animals into the United States and jointly determine data needs to effectively oversee imported animals.

In commenting on a draft of this report, the Departments of Agriculture, Interior and Homeland Security generally agreed with GAO's findings and recommendations. The Department of Health and Human Services provided technical comments only.

What GAO Found

The statutory and regulatory framework for live animal imports has gaps that could allow the introduction of diseases into the United States, according to the experts GAO surveyed, discussions with agency officials, and scientific studies. Specifically,

- The Department of Health and Human Services' Centers for Disease Control and Prevention (CDC) has regulations to prevent the importation of live animals that may pose a previously identified disease risk to humans for some diseases, but gaps in its regulations may allow animals presenting other zoonotic disease risks to enter the United States. CDC has solicited comments in advance of a rulemaking to better prevent the importation of animals that pose zoonotic disease risks.
- The Department of the Interior's Fish and Wildlife Service (FWS) has regulations to prevent imports of nonnative live animals that could become invasive. However, it has not generally emphasized preventing the introduction of disease through importation. FWS is taking some initial steps to address disease risks. For example, in January 2010, the department directed FWS to review statutory authorities and regulations to address existing problems concerning nonnative live animals and recommend tools to better prevent the introduction of new threats.

In contrast, the U.S. Department of Agriculture's Animal and Plant Health Inspection Service (APHIS) has regulations to prevent importing live animals it finds may pose a disease risk to agricultural animals. In 2008, APHIS issued a long-term strategy that would broaden its oversight of live animal imports.

APHIS, the Department of Homeland Security's Customs and Border Protection (CBP), CDC, and FWS have collaborated to meet their responsibilities related to live animal imports by taking actions in five areas—strategic planning, joint strategies, written procedures, leveraging resources, and sharing data.

However, experts GAO surveyed and agency officials GAO interviewed identified barriers to further collaboration on live animal imports, such as different program priorities and unclear roles and responsibilities, which are inherent when multiple agencies have related responsibilities. For example, experts noted that because each of the agencies is focused on a different aspect of live animal imports, no single entity has comprehensive responsibility for the zoonotic and animal disease risks posed by live animal imports.

Experts also reported the need for an entity to help the agencies overcome these barriers to collaboration. Furthermore, the agencies have largely incompatible data systems, and a completion date for CBP's planned data system, which would provide the agencies with full operational access to information on incoming shipments of live animals, has not been established. In addition, APHIS, CBP, CDC, and FWS have yet to jointly determine which data elements on live animal imports are needed in this system for them to effectively oversee these imports, according to CBP officials. As a result, it is unclear whether the data elements in the completed system will meet interagency needs.

ABBREVIATIONS

ACE	Automated Commercial Environment
APHIS	Animal and Plant Health Inspection Service
Bd	*Batrachochytrium dendrobatidis*
CBP	Customs and Border Protection
CDC	Centers for Disease Control and Prevention
DHS	Department of Homeland Security
FWS	Fish and Wildlife Service
ITDS	International Trade Data System
MOU	memorandum of understanding

SARS severe acute respiratory syndrome
USDA U.S. Department of Agriculture

November 8, 2010
The Honorable Joseph I. Lieberman
Chairman

The Honorable Susan M. Collins
Ranking Member

Committee on Homeland Security and
Governmental Affairs
United States Senate

The United States is the world's leading import market for live animals: From 2005 through 2008 more than 1 billion live animals were legally imported into the United States for agriculture, clinical research, education and exhibition, the aquarium and pet industries, and other uses. However, these imports have the potential to transmit zoonotic diseases— infectious diseases that can be transmitted between animals and humans and can cause a substantial number of deaths. Furthermore, zoonotic diseases have represented about 75 percent of newly emerging infectious diseases in recent years. Because of growing international trade and travel, these zoonotic diseases can emerge anywhere and spread rapidly around the globe, as demonstrated by the 2003 outbreak of severe acute respiratory syndrome (SARS), a viral respiratory illness that caused pneumonia in most patients and was responsible for over 700 deaths in East Asia and 43 deaths in Canada. Over the past few years, another zoonotic disease, a highly pathogenic strain of avian influenza, killed millions of wild and domestic birds worldwide and infected over 400 people, more than half of whom died. The spread of zoonotic diseases, as well as other diseases affecting only animals, can take a major economic toll on many industries. For example, the highly pathogenic avian influenza in East Asia cost the affected economies an estimated $10 billion. In the United States, an outbreak of exotic Newcastle disease—a contagious and fatal viral disease affecting birds—resulted in the destruction of over 4.5 million birds in 2002 and 2003 at a cost of more than $395 million in lost trade.

The laws governing the importation of live animals include five statutes that are implemented by four agencies. Specifically,

- *Animal Health Protection Act.* The U.S. Department of Agriculture's (USDA) Animal and Plant Health Inspection Service (APHIS) may prohibit imports of particular animals to prevent the introduction of any pest or disease affecting agricultural animals, such as cattle, horses, poultry, and swine.
- *Lacey Act.* The Department of the Interior's Fish and Wildlife Service (FWS) administers the prohibition against the import of animals that have been individually listed in the statute or prescribed in FWS regulation to be "injurious to human beings, to the interests of agriculture, horticulture, forestry, or to wildlife or the wildlife resources of the United States."
- *The Endangered Species Act of 1973.* FWS administers the prohibition against the import of animals that have been listed as threatened or endangered species and implements other international agreements related to these species.
- *Public Health Service Act.* The Department of Health and Human Services' Centers for Disease Control and Prevention (CDC) issues regulations to prevent the introduction, transmission, and spread of communicable diseases, including zoonotic diseases.
- *Tariff Act of 1930.* The Department of Homeland Security's (DHS) Customs and Border Protection (CBP) is responsible for inspecting imports for compliance with United States law and assisting all federal agencies in enforcing their regulations—including regulations for live animal imports—at ports of entry.

As we have previously reported, when responsibilities cut across more than one federal agency—as they do for the regulation of live animal imports to prevent the introduction and spread of diseases—it is important for agencies to work collaboratively.[1] Taking into account the nation's long-range fiscal challenges, we noted that the federal government must identify ways to deliver results more efficiently and in a way that is consistent with its multiple demands and limited resources. We also identified key practices that can help enhance and sustain federal agencies' collaboration. In addition, we have previously reported on the need to collaborate on animal disease issues. For example, we reported in 2007 on the steps that USDA took to prepare for highly pathogenic avian influenza in poultry and recommended that USDA and DHS clarify their roles during emergency responses to a disease outbreak.[2] Both USDA and DHS officials told us that they have taken preliminary steps to clarify and better define their coordination roles. For example, the two agencies meet on a regular basis to discuss such coordination.

In this context, you asked us to examine (1) potential gaps in the statutory and regulatory framework governing live animal imports, if any, that may allow the introduction and spread of zoonotic and animal diseases; (2) the extent to which APHIS, CBP, CDC, and FWS collaborate to meet their responsibilities and face barriers, if any, to collaboration; and (3) the performance information that the responsible agencies have reported on live animal imports.

To identify potential gaps in the statutory and regulatory framework, we reviewed relevant statutes, the agencies' implementing regulations, and other agency documents. We also reviewed APHIS and FWS data on the number, type, and exporting country of all imported animals regulated by these two agencies for fiscal years 2005 through 2009. For the APHIS and FWS data, we analyzed documentation related to the data, and worked with agency officials to identify data problems, and determined the data were sufficiently reliable for the purposes of providing background to this report. To obtain information on potential gaps in the statutory and regulatory framework as well as agencies' processes for overseeing live animal imports, we interviewed officials at agency headquarters and ports of entry—airports in Atlanta, Baltimore, Los Angeles, New York, and Washington, D.C., and the land border crossings with Mexico at Otay Mesa and San Ysidro, California. At these ports, we focused our review on the legal importation of live animals and not on agencies' actions to prevent animal smuggling. We also reviewed scientific studies on zoonotic and animal diseases, including studies by the National Academies of Sciences.

To examine the extent to which the four agencies collaborate to meet their responsibilities and face barriers, if any, to collaboration, we reviewed each agency's strategic plans, policies, and protocols; reviewed documentation on the allocation of staff resources; and interviewed headquarters officials. We also examined the degree to which the agencies' collaborative efforts reflected the key practices we had identified that can help enhance and sustain collaboration among federal agencies.

To address the first two objectives, we also conducted a two-round survey to identify potential gaps in the current statutory and regulatory framework, how well responsible agencies collaborate to meet their responsibilities, and potential barriers to collaboration. The first round of the survey was conducted from January through February 2010, and the second round was conducted from April through May 2010. We identified knowledgeable experts who had primary employment responsibilities related to or dependent on live animal imports, authored peer-reviewed papers, presented at professional conferences, provided testimony on the subject matter to Congress, or were recognized by their peers as experts on live animal imports. To ensure a cross section of different sectors, we selected experts from federal and state government, academia, nongovernmental organizations, and industry to obtain a broad spectrum of opinions. For the first round, we sent surveys that consisted of open-ended questions (questions that solicit additional information) to our initial list of 39 experts, and we received responses from 33, resulting in a response rate of about 85 percent. On the basis of recommendations provided by those responding in our first round and other experts, we expanded our list of experts to 64 for the survey's second round, which consisted of closed-ended questions (questions with a set of answers to choose from). Of these 64 experts, we received responses from 56, resulting in a response rate of about 88 percent for the second round.

To examine the performance information the responsible agencies have reported on live animal imports in their planning and reporting documents, we reviewed strategic plans, operational plans, mission statements, and annual performance plans and reports from APHIS, CBP, CDC, and FWS. A more detailed discussion of our scope and methodology is presented in appendix I.

We conducted this performance audit from August 2009 through October 2010, in accordance with generally accepted government auditing standards. Those standards require that we plan and perform the audit to obtain sufficient, appropriate evidence to provide a reasonable basis for our findings and conclusions based on our audit objectives. We believe that the evidence obtained provides a reasonable basis for our findings and conclusions based on our audit objectives.

BACKGROUND

APHIS, CBP, CDC, and FWS share responsibility for preventing the importation of live animals that may introduce and spread zoonotic and animal diseases.[3] APHIS, CDC, and FWS have developed regulations that provide specific requirements and restrictions on the importation of animals. In some cases, more than one agency may regulate a given animal. For example, CDC regulates dogs for their risk of spreading rabies to humans, and APHIS regulates dogs from countries with screwworm, a parasite that can cause great damage to domestic livestock and other warm-blooded animals, for their risk of spreading this parasite to agricultural animals. Information on each agency's responsibilities and oversight activities follows and is presented in greater detail in appendix II.

Agencies That Are Responsible for Live Animal Imports

While CBP is responsible for overseeing all imports and assists other agencies in enforcing their import regulations, APHIS, CDC, and FWS have specific statutory and regulatory responsibilities for protecting human, domesticated animal, and wildlife health from risks posed by live animal imports.

APHIS

APHIS restricts the importation of live animals that it has determined may pose a disease risk to agricultural animals, such as cattle, horses, poultry, sheep, and swine. APHIS requires that many of the animals it regulates be visually inspected at the port of entry and generally requires the animals be accompanied by health certificates signed by a licensed veterinarian in the country of export and import permits. APHIS determines the level of inspection for animals on the basis of their associated disease risk, for both the type of animal and country of export. As a result of this determination, APHIS may restrict imports of certain animals from certain countries or require that animals undergo quarantine and disease testing. APHIS veterinarians inspect live animal imports at 15 land ports along the border with Mexico, 20 land ports along the border with Canada, and 30 airports across the continental United States, and in Alaska, Hawaii, and Puerto Rico. In addition, APHIS maintains animal quarantine facilities in southern California, southern Florida, and New York state and oversees private quarantine facilities for birds and horses in southern California. At these quarantine facilities, imported animals are held until test results for various diseases are received.

CBP

CBP assists other federal agencies in enforcing their import regulations, has the primary authority to inspect imports, and seeks to interdict shipments of contraband and the illegal importation of live animals and other products while facilitating the flow of legal travel and trade. According to CBP officials, when a live animal shipment arrives at a port of entry, CBP holds and refers the shipment to the responsible agency or agencies. CBP holds the import until an agency representative is available to release it. After the responsible regulating agency has released the import, CBP clears the import for entry into the United States. CBP staff are present at more than 300 land, air, and sea ports of entry and are trained in the procedures to follow when live animals are presented for customs clearance.

CDC

CDC restricts the importation of live animals that it has determined pose a risk to public health. CDC's restrictions on these imports vary by type of animal and can include banning certain imports, requiring permits, requiring vaccination certificates, and requiring quarantine. CDC staff are not present at all ports of entry to routinely inspect live animal imports. According to CDC officials, CDC relies on APHIS, CBP, and FWS staff to enforce its regulations at ports of entry. When the agencies' staff have questions about enforcing CDC's regulations, they are to contact CDC quarantine public health officers, who are often located at a CDC quarantine station that is at or near the port of entry. CDC has 20 quarantine stations in the continental United States, Alaska, Hawaii, and Puerto Rico.

FWS

FWS restricts the importation of certain wildlife. Specifically, FWS restricts the importation of injurious wildlife and threatened or endangered species and related species for which international trade is regulated under international agreements. Injurious wildlife includes animals that are individually listed in the Lacey Act or prescribed in FWS regulations to be injurious to human beings; to the interests of agriculture, horticulture, or forestry; or to wildlife or the wildlife resources of the United States. FWS seeks to prevent the introduction of invasive species as injurious wildlife under the Lacey Act. Invasive species are alien (or nonnative) species whose introduction does, or is likely to, cause economic or environmental harm or harm to human health.[4] At ports of entry, FWS wildlife inspectors review the required import documents and, for some live animal shipments, perform visual inspections. If FWS determines that the animals are prohibited from importation based on FWS regulations, for example, are injurious to wildlife or threatened or endangered species, it rejects the import unless it has an FWS permit, which may be issued under certain conditions, such as educational purposes. FWS has about 120 wildlife inspectors who handle shipments at 49 ports of entry nationwide, including 7 land ports along the Mexican border, 24 land ports along the Canadian border, and 18 designated ports for air, ocean, rail, and truck across the continental United States and in Alaska and Hawaii.

Number, Type, and Purpose of Live Animals Imports

APHIS and FWS data systems provide information on the number of and purpose for live animal imports, as well as on the country from which the import has been shipped into the United States in recent years.[5] According to the APHIS data system, about 32 million live animals—mostly agricultural or aquacultural—were imported under APHIS regulation in fiscal year 2008, the most recent year for which verified data were available. They included cattle, fish, poultry, and swine. According to the FWS data system, about 177 million live animals—all wildlife—were imported under FWS regulation in fiscal year 2009. About 157 million of these imports were fish. Other types of animals imported under FWS regulation included amphibians, birds, corals, crustaceans, insects, mammals, mollusks, and reptiles. More information about the number and type of live animal imports is in appendix III.

Interagency Collaboration

In 2000, we reported that agencies face a range of barriers when they attempt to collaborate with other agencies.[6] With these barriers in place, federal agencies carry out programs in a fragmented, uncoordinated way, resulting in a patchwork of programs that can waste scarce funds, confuse and frustrate program customers, and limit the overall effectiveness of the federal effort. Subsequently, in 2005, we identified key practices that can help enhance and sustain collaboration among federal agencies.[7] Among the practices we identified were (1) defining and articulating a common outcome; (2) defining and agreeing on roles and responsibilities; (3) establishing mutually reinforcing or joint strategies; (4) identifying and addressing needs by leveraging resources; and (5) establishing compatible policies, procedures, and other means to operate across agency boundaries. In our 2005 report, we stated that while we generally believe that the application of as many of these practices as possible increases the likelihood of effective collaboration, we also recognize that there is a wide range of situations and circumstances in which agencies work together.

The One Health Initiative Discusses Collaboration to Address Zoonotic and Animal Diseases

Recognizing that zoonotic and animal diseases are interconnected, several organizations—including the American Medical Association, the American Veterinary Medical Association, and CDC—have taken steps to support the One Health concept, which is a worldwide strategy for expanding interdisciplinary collaboration and communications in all aspects of health care for humans and animals. In 2007, the American Veterinary Medical Association established the One Health Initiative Task Force to study the feasibility of a campaign to facilitate collaboration and cooperation among health science professions, academic institutions, governmental agencies, and industries to help, among other things, assess, treat, and prevent cross-species disease transmission. In 2008, the task force framed the issue, stating that the convergence of people, animals, and the environment has created a new dynamic in which the health of each group is inextricably interconnected.[8] Examples of recent diseases causing animal, human, environmental, or economic harm are described in appendix IV.

The National Invasive Species Council Focuses on Collaboration among Federal Agencies

In 1999, an executive order established the National Invasive Species Council, cochaired by the Secretaries of Agriculture, Commerce, and the Interior.[9] Its members are the Secretaries and Administrators of 13 federal departments and agencies. The council was charged with providing national leadership; seeing that the federal invasive species activities are coordinated, complementary, cost-efficient, and effective; and encouraging planning and action at local, tribal, state, and regional levels. The range of invasive species issues that the council is attempting to address includes live animal imports that may bring diseases into the United States. The executive order also required the Secretary of the Interior to establish the Invasive Species Advisory Committee, a group of 30 nonfederal stakeholders from diverse constituencies (representing state, tribal, local, and private concerns) around the nation, to advise the council on invasive species issues. In 2008, the council issued its most recent management plan for invasive species, the *2008-2012 National Invasive Species Management Plan.* The management plan lists goals and performance elements that identify the federal agency with the lead or participant role. It includes tasks pertaining to pathogens or diseases. For example, one of the tasks is to develop a process for identifying high-priority invasive plants, animals, and plant or animal pathogens for agencies' actions. The council is currently preparing a progress report on the implementation of the 2008-through-2012 plan, with an expected completion date of October 2010.

Recent Studies Have Discussed the Regulation of Live Animal Imports

Studies by the National Academies of Sciences and others have found significant deficiencies in the regulation of live animal imports that may allow the introduction and spread of emerging zoonotic and animal diseases. For example,

A 2005 National Academies of Sciences report referred to a "patchwork of federal policies and agencies with limited or ill-defined jurisdiction" for the importation of wildlife, "a significant gap in preventing and rapidly detecting emergent diseases," and "a lack of coordinated federal oversight" over disease issues associated with these animals.[10] It found that wildlife are imported daily with little or no health monitoring, increasing the likelihood that zoonotic or animal diseases will enter the United States. The report also noted that the animal health infrastructure "does not have formal and comprehensive-based science and risk analysis systems for anticipating potential challenges to animal health; ranking their likelihood of occurring and likely severity; evaluating alternative prevention, detection, and diagnostic systems; and using this information to make appropriate policy decisions."

- A 2007 study by the Defenders of Wildlife, a nonprofit organization that supports wildlife conservation, concluded that no law mandates a comprehensive assessment of the potential risk from the importation of a given nonnative species to human and animal health.[11]
- In the November 2009 issue of CDC's journal, *Emerging Infectious Diseases,* scientists reported on their study of mammal imports and concluded that these imports provide numerous opportunities for zoonotic pathogens to enter the United States. The study recommended increased surveillance of imported animals that pose an increased risk of harboring zoonotic pathogens.[12]

Gaps in the Statutory and Regulatory Framework for Some Live Animal Imports May Contribute to Disease Risks, according to Experts and Agency Officials

The statutory and regulatory framework governing live animal imports has gaps that could allow the introduction and spread of zoonotic diseases and diseases affecting wildlife, according to the experts we surveyed, our discussions with agency officials, and scientific studies on zoonotic and animal diseases. In particular, while APHIS has regulations in place to protect agricultural animals from the risk of diseases in live animal imports, CDC does not fully use its statutory authority to prevent the importation of live animals that may pose a risk of zoonotic diseases, and FWS generally does not restrict the entry of imported wildlife that may pose disease risks.

APHIS Has Regulations to Protect U.S. Agriculture from Live Animal Imports That Could Carry Disease

APHIS has regulations to prevent the importation of live animals that it has determined could pose a disease risk to agricultural animals. For example, APHIS requires that commercial birds, such as those imported for resale, breeding, or public display from countries other than Canada be quarantined until found free of evidence of communicable diseases of poultry. In addition, APHIS restricts the importation of certain animals from certain countries, such as cattle from countries where foot-and-mouth disease—a highly contagious viral disease of cloven-hoofed animals such as cattle, swine, and sheep—has been detected.

USDA's Office of Inspector General has performed several audits of APHIS's live animal import processes in recent years. For example, an August 2010 audit report identified weaknesses in the procedures APHIS used to handle animals destined for a quarantine facility, beginning with the precautions it took when receiving the animals into the country and continuing to the conditions at the quarantine facilities.[13] According to the report, APHIS officials did not identify these weaknesses because they did not exercise sufficient oversight to ensure import and quarantine requirements were met. Instead, they relied on the experience and expertise of port staff and import center officials. In addition, a 2008 audit report on APHIS's controls over live animal imports indicated that APHIS relies on health certificates from the exporting country to certify the animal's health condition, age, and other import requirements.[14] However, the report stated, APHIS does not have adequate processes to determine whether individual problems detected represent a larger systemic noncompliance that needs to be addressed by agency inspection personnel or the exporting country. The Inspector General recommended that APHIS establish an automated system of records to document and track problems with live imported animals and report these problems to key stakeholders.

Table 1. Overview of Federal Agencies' Disease Risk Screening for Selected Types of Imported Animals

Type of imported animal	Regulating agency[a]	Disease testing at quarantine facility	Assessment by U.S. agency of disease presence in exporting country	Health certificate from exporting country	Visual inspection at U.S. ports of entry for disease
Cattle from Canada or Mexico[b]	APHIS	c	APHIS	APHIS	APHIS
Commercial birds not from Canada	APHIS FWS	APHIS	APHIS	APHIS	APHIS
Rodents from Africa	CDC FWS	c	CDC[d]	c	FWS[e]
Rodents not from Africa	FWS	c	c	c	c
Amphibians	FWS	c	c	c	c

Source: APHIS, CDC, and FWS regulations and guidance and discussions with agency officials.

Note: FWS does not screen shipments of live animals for disease risk, with the exception of imported salmon. FWS requires that all carriers transporting wild mammals and birds to the United States have a certificate of veterinary medical inspection signed by a veterinarian.

[a]CBP does not develop regulations for how to import an animal, so it is not included in the list of regulating agencies.

[b]Cattle from Mexico are tested for tuberculosis and brucellosis and checked for ticks prior to entry into the United States.

[c]APHIS, FWS, and CDC do not perform this screening process for this imported animal.

[d]In 2003, CDC restricted the importation of rodents from Africa based on concerns about monkeypox.

[e]FWS inspects shipments of rodents from Africa to assess if the rodents are in compliance with CDC regulations.

According to the Inspector General, APHIS planned to implement this recommendation and to have officials analyze data from the system each month and communicate with stakeholders regarding corrective actions. According to agency officials, APHIS began using this system—the Veterinary Services Process Streamlining System—in June 2010.

We found that the agency has screening processes in place for the imported animals it regulates that generally do not exist for other imported animals regulated by other agencies. For example, as table 1 shows, for cattle from Canada or Mexico, APHIS is to assess whether key diseases are present in the prospective exporting country, require a health certificate from a veterinarian in the exporting country, and visually inspect the cattle. In addition, for cattle not from Canada, Mexico, Central America, or the West Indies, APHIS requires that the cattle be quarantined to determine that they are free from disease. As the table shows, CDC and FWS do not generally have similar processes for the animals they regulate. (See app. V for additional types of imported animals and federal agency disease risk screening requirements.)

Although APHIS does not regulate the importation of all live animals, most of the experts responding to our survey supported a broader role for APHIS. (See apps. VI and VII for more details on these experts and their responses to the survey.) Specifically,

- Fifty-three of the 55 experts responding to our survey question about APHIS's statutory and regulatory framework indicated that changes are needed to prevent the importation of zoonotic and animal diseases.
- Forty eight of the 54 experts responding to a question in our survey strongly or somewhat supported giving APHIS the authority to consider the disease risk from wildlife as part of its existing risk assessment process.

In 2008, APHIS took a step toward broadening its oversight of live animal imports and becoming more responsive to emerging disease threats. It issued a long-term strategy—known as VS2015—that identifies key changes APHIS states are essential for the organization in 2015, including (1) an expanded veterinary health mission and (2) an increased focus on disease prevention, preparedness, detection, and early response activities.[15] Specifically, *Expanded veterinary health mission.* Consistent with the One Health concept, APHIS would expand its mission to address not only disease issues that affect agricultural animals but also those associated with zoonotic and wildlife diseases. According to the long-term strategy, APHIS plans to

- provide national leadership on the animal health component associated with public health,
- work with wildlife entities to address health issues that affect production agriculture and wildlife health, and
- lend its veterinary assets (e.g., laboratory networks, stockpiles, and response corps) and provide leadership in areas within its expertise (e.g., epidemiology, surveillance, planning, risk analysis, and modeling) when public health issues arise involving nonnative and wildlife species.

Increased focus on disease prevention, preparedness, detection, and early response activities. APHIS's goal is to reduce the frequency of disease outbreaks that affect animals by emphasizing prevention and preparedness. According to the long-term strategy, APHIS plans to

- design and direct comprehensive national animal health surveillance systems capable of finding foreign, emerging, and known diseases, and of supporting international reporting and trade verification requirements;
- investigate potential emerging animal health threats and apply decision criteria to determine appropriate early responses;
- when needed, extend its prevention and early response efforts to address animal health issues occurring outside of the United States, including identifying, prioritizing, planning, and directing APHIS-funded animal health surveillance and disease control or eradication programs carried out overseas; and
- assist other countries as they develop their animal health capacities and provide leadership in the development of global animal health standards and methods.

In support of VS2015, APHIS formed an internal work team that, according to agency officials, is working on more comprehensive training of APHIS staff; better use of technology for collaboration, communication, and data tracking; and the engagement of industry as a more active partner.

CDC Has Regulations for Some Live Animal Imports but Does Not Prevent the Importation of Many Animals That May Pose a Risk of Zoonotic Diseases

CDC has regulations to prevent the importation of certain live animals that may pose a previously identified disease risk to humans for some diseases, such as rabies, but, according to agency officials, CDC's regulations are limited to specific species and regions and do not comprehensively prevent the importation of animals that are known to present a high risk of zoonotic diseases. That is, CDC restricts imports of some animals to prevent the introduction of specific diseases: nonhuman primates, to prevent the spread of tuberculosis, among other things; bats, to prevent the introduction of a variety of infectious pathogens, including *Ebola* virus; rodents from Africa, to prevent monkeypox; dogs and cats, to prevent zoonotic diseases in general and rabies in dogs; and certain turtles, to prevent *Salmonella.* In 2004, CDC banned the importation of birds from specified countries based on the threat that imports from such countries increased the risk that highly pathogenic avian influenza may be introduced into the United States. In 2009, CDC rescinded this ban. According to CDC's notice rescinding the ban, APHIS's import restrictions on birds and poultry adequately address risks to human health, and CDC will work closely with APHIS to monitor the international situation regarding highly pathogenic avian influenza.

Even though CDC has these restrictions, imported animals that present a zoonotic risk could enter into the United States. For example,

- While CDC generally requires proof of current rabies vaccination and the confinement of most dogs for up to 30 days after vaccination, it has received reports of large-volume shipments of puppies intended for immediate resale. According to agency officials, these animals often appear younger than the age on their accompanying documents, that is, they are too young to receive an effective rabies vaccination, and their vaccination status is questionable. In addition, according to agency officials, if CDC finds at ports of entry that a dog was not vaccinated for rabies, the agency allows it to enter, if the owner agrees to keep the dog confined until it can be properly vaccinated and then confined for an additional 30 days following vaccination to prevent the potential spread of rabies. However, state and local agencies that are to monitor confinement frequently lack resources to do so, according to CDC officials.

- CDC's regulations do not require rabies vaccinations for cats, which are highly susceptible to certain strains of rabies virus and can also transmit the infection to humans.

In addition, experts responding to our survey told us that CDC generally reacts only when a zoonotic disease problem arises. For example, since the 1970s it has been well known that monkeypox, a zoonotic disease, was endemic to Africa. However, according CDC officials, CDC did not have a process to conduct a risk assessment on the potential movement of monkeypox to the United States. Furthermore, they said, if such a risk assessment process had been in place, CDC might have restricted the importation of certain animals from Africa. After a 2003 outbreak of monkeypox in the United States, which sickened over 70 people, CDC restricted the importation of African rodents and other animals that may carry the monkeypox virus. However, CDC still allows the importation of rodents from countries outside of Africa, and these imported rodents are not subject to examination to determine whether they may be carrying zoonotic disease. Furthermore, according to experts responding to our survey and CDC officials, the importation of many other wildlife species is allowed with little or no screening for zoonotic disease risks. For example, mice, rats, and gerbils are not screened for zoonotic diseases, but the animal family that includes these animals has been found to harbor 21 zoonotic diseases.

CDC's regulation of live animal imports does not sufficiently protect against zoonotic disease risks, according to the experts responding to our survey and scientific studies. According to 50 of the 55 experts responding to our survey question about CDC's statutory and regulatory framework, changes are needed. For example, 40 of the 51 experts responding to a question in our survey strongly or somewhat supported giving CDC the authority to use pre-import screening, such as a process that assesses disease risk by species and country and determines allowable imports on the basis of that assessment. CDC is considering other regulatory mechanisms that would allow CDC to suspend the entry of animal imports into the United States from designated foreign countries for public health reasons. Decisions to suspend animal imports from designated foreign countries would be based on the existence of a communicable disease in that country and the likelihood that allowing such imports would increase the likelihood of introducing disease into the United States. While these regulatory mechanisms are not specifically "pre-import screening," these mechanisms may serve the same purpose.

The CDC officials we interviewed acknowledged gaps in the agency's regulation of live animal imports for zoonotic diseases. To address this problem, in 2007, CDC issued an advance notice of proposed rulemaking on live animal imports to take steps to better prevent the introduction of zoonotic disease into the United States. The questions raised in the advance notice of proposed rulemaking include whether CDC should (1) establish a regulation that maintains a list of species or categories of high-risk animals for which importation is restricted (e.g., either prohibited from entry or subject to certain requirements), (2) apply these potential restrictions to broad taxonomic groupings (e.g., all rodents) or individual species, (3) issue these potential restrictions on a limited geographical basis (i.e., certain countries or regions) or more broadly, and (4) make rabies vaccination a requirement for entry into the United States for all dogs and cats. CDC is currently analyzing the comments that it received, revising the proposed language, and conducting economic analyses. CDC expects to publish a notice of proposed rulemaking in 2011.

Although FWS Has Regulations for Injurious Wildlife, It Does Not Restrict the Entry of Imported Wildlife That May Pose Disease Risks

Under the authority of the Lacey Act, FWS has implemented regulations to restrict imports of various types of nonnative live animals that have been identified as injurious wildlife because, for example, they could become invasive.[16] However, FWS's regulations allow other types of wildlife to enter the United States with little assessment of the disease risk or health status of the animal, despite the possible presence of diseases in animals that are not endemic to the United States.

For example, FWS does not restrict the importation of live amphibians or assess their risk for the presence of disease, creating a risk that the Bd fungus (*Batrachochytrium dendrobatidis*)—which causes a highly contagious disease that is potentially fatal to amphibians—will continue to enter and spread. The Department of the Interior has been petitioned by the Defenders of Wildlife to ban imports of live amphibians unless they are free of the Bd pathogen.

As of September 2010, the department planned to gather information from the public before deciding whether to develop a regulation in response to this petition. Furthermore, the Lacey Act's process to ban the importation of injurious wildlife often requires too much time for the process to be effective, according to FWS officials and experts responding to our survey. On average, it takes about 4 years for FWS to identify a species or group of species as injurious wildlife. During this time, the animals in question continue to be imported into the United States.

In addition, according to FWS officials, FWS inspectors visually inspect some live wildlife imports, which may include observation for signs of disease, but they are not veterinarians, and they do not have expertise in detecting diseased animals.

Furthermore, experts responding to our survey said that visual inspections have limited effectiveness in detecting diseased animals. They noted that it is often difficult to distinguish between a healthy, uninfected animal and an apparently healthy but infected animal, and even healthy animals can carry pathogens that could harm other species or humans but not harm the host.

In written comments to our survey, some experts reported that the Lacey Act should be amended to better prevent the importation of live animals that pose disease risks, while other experts said FWS should use its current authority to improve its regulations in this area.

According to 52 of the 55 experts responding to our survey question about FWS's statutory and regulatory framework, changes are needed. Of the 53 experts who responded to our survey questions about specific potential changes, 44 strongly or somewhat supported giving FWS the authority to use pre-import screening, and 43 strongly or somewhat supported having FWS expedite the process for classifying species as injurious wildlife.

The Department of the Interior has taken preliminary steps that may address gaps in FWS's regulation of live animal imports. In addition to reviewing the petition to restrict amphibian imports, in January 2010, the Secretary of the Interior directed FWS to comprehensively review statutory authorities and regulations to address existing invasive species problems and to recommend potential tools to more effectively prevent the introduction of new invasive threats.

According to Department of the Interior testimony provided at a March 2010 hearing on invasive species, FWS is reviewing several proposals to create a more proactive and comprehensive approach to preventing the spread of invasive species, including streamlining the evaluation process, examining gaps that the Lacey Act's injurious wildlife provisions leave in the listing process, revising its risk assessment process, and supporting improved regulatory and educational approaches.[17]

AGENCIES HAVE COLLABORATED TO MEET THEIR RESPONSIBILITIES, BUT EXPERTS AND AGENCY OFFICIALS IDENTIFIED BARRIERS TO FURTHER COLLABORATION

APHIS, CBP, CDC, and FWS have collaborated to meet their responsibilities by taking actions in five areas—strategic planning, joint strategies, written procedures, leveraging resources, and sharing data— but experts responding to our survey and agency officials we interviewed identified barriers to further collaboration on live animal imports. As we have previously reported, agencies encounter a range of barriers when they attempt to collaborate with other agencies.[18] Experts also identified the need for an entity to help the agencies overcome these barriers.

Although Agencies Have Collaborated to Meet Common Goals, They Face Barriers to Additional Collaboration

Strategic planning. APHIS, CBP, CDC, and FWS have engaged in strategic planning that recognizes the need for joint efforts to reduce the risks of zoonotic and animal diseases from live animal imports. Specifically, according to APHIS's 2007-through-2012 strategic plan, it is working with CBP to reduce pest and disease threats at the borders. The strategic plan also states that the agency's risk assessment protocols must recognize the growing importance of zoonotic diseases and the need to work with public health agencies to reduce the risk of these diseases. Within APHIS, the program office of Veterinary Services' strategic plan—VS2015—states that Veterinary Services intends to meet future animal health challenges, such as emerging zoonotic and animal diseases, by 2015. According to this plan, Veterinary Services will expand its mission to include public health concerns connected to any type of animal. In addition, the plan states that Veterinary Services will work with wildlife entities to address health issues that affect the health of both agricultural animals and wildlife. Such collaboration would involve working with CDC and FWS. According to CBP's strategic plan for 2009 through 2014, CBP is actively pursuing new relationships with CDC to enhance CBP's response to public health threats. CDC officials told us that it has identified a strategic goal to enhance CDC's ability to prevent, detect, and respond to zoonotic diseases associated with the importation of live animals.[19]

Furthermore, according to FWS's law enforcement strategic plan for 2006 through 2010, increased coordination will be required with agencies (such as CDC and APHIS) that are responsible for addressing linkages between wildlife trade and the cross-border spread of zoonotic and animal diseases.

As we have previously reported, federal agencies can use their strategic and annual performance plans as tools to drive collaboration with other agencies and partners and establish complementary goals and strategies for achieving results.[20] While the agencies' strategic planning addresses some concerns about the disease risk from live imported animals, it does not specify how they will collaborate to address the risk of disease from live animal imports. Such specificity is difficult, according to several experts responding to our survey, in part because the agencies' program priorities are based on different missions, constituencies, and priorities. In particular, experts responding to our survey noted that because each of the agencies is focused on a different aspect of live animal imports, no single entity has comprehensive responsibility for the zoonotic and animal diseases risks posed by live animal imports. As one expert noted, the principal barrier to collaboration is agencies' "failure to take a broader view of the entire importation process," focusing instead on only those components of the process each agency controls under its statutory authority. As we have previously reported, when agencies do not have a compelling rationale, such as legislation, directives, or their perceptions of the benefits from collaboration, it is difficult to overcome differences in missions and priorities and to define and articulate a common outcome that is consistent with their respective agency missions.[21] However, as the One Health concept recognizes, human and animal diseases are interconnected. In this regard, the federal agencies that are responsible for live animal imports appear to have a common goal—preventing the introduction and spread of zoonotic and animal diseases from live animal imports.

Joint strategies to reduce disease risk from imported live animals. Several of the agencies we reviewed participated in joint strategies to directly or indirectly address risks posed by imported live animals. For example,

- APHIS, FWS, and the Department of Commerce's National Oceanic and Atmospheric Administration jointly developed the *National Aquatic Animal Health Plan* in 2008.[22] Under this plan, the agencies are to prepare coordinated research and development strategies and budget recommendations to provide a framework for how the three agencies should develop programs for diseases that affect the health of aquatic animals, including finfish, crustaceans, and mollusks.[23] Activities addressed in the plan include (1) defining pathogens of national concern; (2) preventing, controlling, and managing pathogens or the diseases caused by those pathogens; (3) describing and implementing surveillance programs; and (4) describing strategies for continued outreach and awareness regarding national aquatic animal health strategies and the plan. As of July 2010, an advisory committee was being formed and a surveillance network had been established for viral hemorrhagic septicemia, a deadly infectious fish disease that affects 28 susceptible species of fresh and saltwater fish and is a growing threat in the Great Lakes region. While this plan is not fully launched, experts responding to our survey commented that the effort has strengthened collaboration among international, federal, and state partners. According to the Department of the Interior, this plan is a model for federal cooperation with regard to movement of aquatic animal diseases, and it will be broadened to include amphibians and reptiles in the future.

- The National Invasive Species Council's *2008-2012 National Invasive Species Management Plan*, which is the council's primary coordination tool for the prevention and control of invasive species, includes an objective to expand the coordination of invasive species programs and expenditures to leverage resources. It also directs the relevant agencies to update the budget for federal agencies' expenditures concerning invasive species. The council expects to report on the plan's progress in October 2010. APHIS, CBP, and FWS have participated in the council since its inception, while CDC has recently rejoined the group.
- The Aquatic Nuisance Species Task Force—an intergovernmental organization composed of 13 federal agencies, including FWS, APHIS, and the Department of Commerce's National Oceanic and Atmospheric Administration—is working to prevent and control aquatic nuisance species.[24] The task force was established by the Nonindigenous Aquatic Nuisance Prevention and Control Act of 1990.[25] In 2007, the task force developed a strategic plan for 2007 through 2012 that includes an objective for analyzing and evaluating rapid response plans, including plans for foreign animal disease events, to see how they could apply to reported introductions of invasive species. In addition, the task force and the National Invasive Species Council have identified various pathways by which pathogens can be introduced into the country. These pathways include container

water in which aquatic animals are transported. According to FWS officials, this container water can contain pathogens and, in some instances, importers may not disinfect the water before disposing of it.

- In 2009, APHIS, CBP, CDC, and several southern California animal agencies formed a task force to address issues with the importation of puppies, such as reducing and eliminating the illegal smuggling and selling of dogs that are underage, in poor health, or do not have the required health certifications.

These strategies are positive steps toward furthering the common goal of preventing disease risk from live animal imports. As we have previously reported, collaborating agencies need to establish strategies that work in concert with those of their partners or are joint in nature.[26] Such strategies help in aligning the partner agencies' activities, core processes, and resources to accomplish the common outcome. In addition, all 56 experts responding to our survey indicated that it is very or moderately important for the federal agencies to collaborate to develop a coordinated national strategy to better align activities, processes, and resources.

According to the experts responding to our survey, the agencies develop joint strategies to respond quickly to emergencies as they arise, but the agencies tend to develop joint strategies in reaction to an identified problem, rather than in anticipation of it. For example, one expert noted that the outbreak of monkeypox in 2003 spread to prairie dogs and subsequently to humans. The expert, as well as CDC officials, commented that although this outbreak was addressed promptly, it might have been avoided if officials had considered the risk of this disease and taken appropriate actions before an outbreak occurred.

Several studies and CDC officials also cited the need for a formal joint strategy to prevent the introduction of zoonotic and animal diseases, such as a comprehensive risk assessment system, and for responding to health risks, such as having plans and resources for early detection and response. Experts also commented that the development of such a system should focus on how live animal imports affect the health of humans, agricultural animals, and wildlife. Moreover, the 2005 National Academies of Sciences report noted that the animal health infrastructure does not have formal and comprehensive science-based risk analysis systems for anticipating potential challenges to animal health. In addition, experts responding to our survey commented that a comprehensive risk assessment system should be established on the basis of an analysis of imported animals to assess the threat that these animals pose. The experts stated that the components of this risk assessment system might include an analysis of the species' exporting country, diseases of concern, typical packaging and delivery times, and methods of shipment of concern, among other things. Suggested uses of the risk assessment include targeting passengers and cargo most likely to be carrying prohibited animals, and making decisions based on this information. According to experts responding to our survey, agencies could use this information to determine whether the importation of particular species from certain countries should be banned and which animals require pre-import screening, including the increased use of disease testing and quarantine at the ports of entry. For example, such risk assessment could be similar to APHIS's process, which assesses the disease risk within defined regions on a consistent and scientific basis and evaluates the animal health status of countries or regions requesting approval to import live animals into the United States.

Written procedures for ports of entry. The four agencies have written procedures to follow when working with other federal agencies at ports of entry. In particular, three of the agencies—APHIS, CBP, and FWS—signed a memorandum of understanding (MOU) on forfeiture that lays out the specific roles and responsibilities each has for seizing, quarantining, and disposing of birds that are brought into the United States in violation of laws or regulations. In addition, APHIS and CBP signed an MOU that outlines the agencies' roles for entry and inspection of the imported animals that APHIS regulates. Two of the four agencies—APHIS and CBP—also have other types of written procedures, while CDC is developing guidance, according to CDC officials. Specifically,

- APHIS has guidance that outlines the procedures and responsibilities that its division of Veterinary Services is to follow with CBP in handling legally and illegally imported pet and performing birds arriving as passenger baggage, from when the birds arrive at the port of entry until they are released to enter into the United States or refused entry. For example, the guidance specifies which birds are eligible for entry and which agency is responsible for (1) transferring birds to a quarantine station and (2) obtaining supplies for handling the birds.
- CBP has a standard operating procedure that informs its staff at ports of entry of procedures to follow in handling shipments of APHIS-regulated live fish. Specifically, if the species has been approved by APHIS for import, CBP staff are to allow it to proceed; if the species

has not already been approved, then the staff are to hold the shipment for Veterinary Services; if the species is not regulated by APHIS, CBP is to hold the shipment for USDA's Agricultural Marketing Service, which administers programs that facilitate the marketing of U.S. agricultural products.

- CBP and APHIS have written guidance for coordinating their processing of live animals arriving at Canadian land border ports of entry.
- CBP and APHIS have written procedures for the importation of livestock at four Mexican land border ports of entry and certain cattle at all Mexican land border ports of entry.
- CBP has written procedures to help its port staff make appropriate referrals to other agencies.
- According to CDC officials, the agency is developing internal standard operating procedures to distribute to its staff at ports of entry on CDC-regulated animals. The officials said the first such guidance will be on how to handle imported turtles, although the officials did not know when this guidance would be issued.

While the agencies have developed some written procedures, officials told us that they do not have written procedures for all animal imports. In the absence of written procedures, agencies collaborate informally at ports of entry on how to handle incoming shipments. Specifically, according to FWS headquarters officials we spoke with, FWS and CDC port officials regularly coordinate on physical inspections of live animals they both regulate, such as nonhuman primates, turtles and tortoises, and bats. For example, according to CBP officials, when turtles are imported into the United States, CBP usually contacts FWS inspectors. According to FWS officials, if the type of turtle being imported is not banned, FWS may contact CDC or APHIS for inspection or further action if it believes there is potential for another type of violation, such as undersized turtles that pose a risk for *Salmonella* (CDC) or turtles with ticks that may have Heartwater infection (APHIS), a potentially fatal disease to cattle. In addition, officials at ports of entry from CBP and APHIS told us that they usually have access to an official from another agency to speak with if questions arise about a shipment. For example, CBP officials at several ports told us they contact APHIS, CDC, and FWS officials informally through e-mails, telephone calls, and in person in order to verify that procedures are being followed for live animal imports they regulate. Finally, some experts responding to our survey noted that officials at some ports have cultivated effective collaborative relationships. However, we have previously reported that by using informal coordination mechanisms, agencies may rely on relationships with individual officials to ensure effective collaboration and that these informal relationships could end once personnel move to their next assignments.[27] Without written procedures, agencies' roles and responsibilities are not clearly defined. We reported that agencies can strengthen their commitment to work collaboratively by articulating their roles and responsibilities in formal documents to facilitate decision making. Such formal documents can include MOUs, interagency guidance, or interagency planning documents, signed by senior officials in the respective agencies. These documents can clarify which agencies will be responsible for particular activities, and how they will organize their joint and individual efforts. Experts responding to our survey generally agreed that uncertainty about agencies' roles and responsibilities for imported animals is a barrier, particularly for species that are (1) not regulated for disease risk by any agency or (2) regulated by more than one agency. For example, several of the experts noted that federal regulations do not address the risk to human and animal health posed by the importation of most nonnative wild animals, such as non-African rodents, and that where regulations do allow for the import of nonnative wild animals, no disease assessment is made. In addition, the agencies do not have written procedures for all species that are regulated by more than one agency, such as reptiles. For example, APHIS and FWS do not have a written procedure to coordinate their shared responsibilities for regulating reptiles—which are a source of *Salmonella* infection in humans and also carry disease-causing parasites.

Leveraging resources. APHIS, CBP, CDC, and FWS have taken steps to leverage resources—staff and funding—to enhance their ability to address disease risks associated with live animal imports. For example,

- APHIS has provided CDC headquarters with a liaison to represent USDA's interests on a broad range of topics, including live animal imports, and shares information with CDC on zoonotic diseases. CDC officials stated that they are currently exploring the possibility of establishing a DHS liaison.
- APHIS, FWS, the U.S. Coast Guard, and the Department of Commerce's National Oceanic and Atmospheric Administration worked together to launch two national campaigns designed to help the public understand its role in preventing the introduction and spread of zoonotic and animal diseases. The first campaign, called

"Stop Aquatic Hitchhikers," is directed toward the public who engage in aquatic activities to, among other things, prevent the spread of invasive species, zoonotic diseases, and animal pathogens. The second campaign, "Habitattitude," is directed toward, among others, pet owners to promote environmentally friendly behaviors, such as not releasing nonnative pets into the environment.

While the agencies have worked together to leverage their resources, they do not separate the amount of funding and level of staff for live animal imports from other agency activities.[28] As a result, they may not be able to determine whether their funding and staff are sufficient, and the extent to which they could be leveraged in a collaborative effort. Furthermore, the four agencies vary significantly in the extent to which they have resources for regulating live animal imports, according to agency officials and experts responding to our survey. For example, APHIS has staff who perform services—such as review of information provided by foreign governments—to support assessments of the risk of live animal imports into the United States. In addition, APHIS has quarantine facilities that inspect and test imports for diseases prior to an animal being released into the United States. In contrast, FWS does not have similar resources for assessing risk and has no quarantine facilities. The experts responding to our survey also noted that resource constraints, such as limited facilities and staff, make it difficult for the four agencies to devote enough time to collaboration when they face time constraints in completing daily tasks. The experts responding to our survey noted that under these conditions it is challenging for the agencies to collaborate. As we have previously reported, collaborating agencies should identify the human, information technology, physical, and financial resources needed to initiate or sustain their collaborative effort.[29] By assessing their relative strengths and limitations, collaborating agencies can look for opportunities to obtain additional benefits that would not be available if they were working separately. Forty-nine of the 54 experts who responded to a survey question about leveraging resources strongly or somewhat supported leveraging APHIS resources to assist FWS in preventing the importation of animal diseases, and 48 indicated that APHIS resources should be leveraged to assist CDC in preventing the importation of zoonotic diseases. In addition, according to APHIS officials we spoke with, APHIS has expertise that could assist FWS and CDC in assessing disease risks in other countries. Furthermore, 50 of 56 experts responding to our survey reported that it is very or moderately important for federal agencies to collaborate to develop a plan to maximize existing resources.

Data sharing. As we have reported, agencies can facilitate collaboration by coordinating data information systems for carrying out shared objectives.[30] According to CBP officials, the agency is developing the International Trade Data System (ITDS) within the Automated Commercial Environment (ACE) system. ACE will serve as a Web-based portal for exchanging trade information among federal agencies that share the responsibility for facilitating international trade.[31] Currently, APHIS and FWS can access data, such as importer data and other related information, but cannot enter information into the system. In its *2009 Report to Congress on the International Trade Data System,* CBP stated that agencies participating in ITDS, including APHIS, CDC, and FWS, have formed working groups to ensure, among other things, that data elements are identified and specified to the detail necessary in shipment information. For example, according to agency officials, a working group of agencies that use data on or oversee imported eggs was formed. While agencies do not yet have access to an integrated data system, agency officials and experts responding to our survey identified efforts to share data. For example, FWS has shared its data with CDC to identify possible health risks from imports of nonnative wildlife. In addition, according to APHIS officials, the agency is beginning to implement terminology in its trade database that is consistent with CBP's so that the agencies can share information about incoming shipments. According to CBP officials, APHIS, CDC, FWS and other agencies will ultimately be able to enter and retrieve information using the ACE system. However, CBP officials do not have a target date for when APHIS, CBP, CDC, and FWS would have full operational access to ACE, and they stated that a unified data system has been a goal since 1995; ITDS has been ongoing since 2006. In addition, while the agencies participating in ITDS have formed workgroups for some types of trade data, APHIS, CBP, CDC, and FWS have yet to jointly determine which data elements are needed for them to effectively oversee live animal imports, according to CBP officials. As a result, it is unclear whether the data in the completed system will meet interagency needs. Until ITDS is completed, the agencies responsible for live animal imports continue to collect and rely on data that are not easily shared. Experts responding to our survey pointed out that the agencies have not linked their data systems so that they can share information on live animal shipments, as well as track violations. In particular, APHIS and FWS maintain separate databases that contain information on shipments of animals that they regulate, and CBP maintains a database on all imports, including live animals. However, the three databases do not interface, so that agencies regulating the same shipment of live animals can have access to the same information at the same time.

Experts Responding to Our Survey Identified the Need for an Entity to Help the Agencies Overcome Barriers to Collaboration

The experts responding to our survey, including federal and state agency officials, also generally pointed to the need for some formal entity to help overcome barriers to achieving their common interest in preventing the importation of animals that may be carrying zoonotic or animal diseases. For example, one expert observed that such an entity could help the agencies identify gaps and inconsistencies in the overall regulation of live animal imports for zoonotic and animal diseases and enable the agencies to collaborate regularly, and 53 of 56 experts responding to our survey reported that it was very or moderately important for the agencies to collaborate to identify gaps in regulations related to live animal imports. We asked the experts about the extent to which they would support the creation of a workgroup to help the federal agencies collaborate in preventing the importation of animals that may be carrying zoonotic and animal diseases. Most of the experts responding to this question—52 of 55—strongly or somewhat supported the creation of such a workgroup. (See app. VII for the experts' detailed responses.)

APHIS, CDC, and FWS Have Reported Some Information on Their Performance on Live Animal Imports

APHIS and FWS routinely report information on their performance to oversee the importation of live animals, and CDC has reported performance information for one species. CBP does not report any performance information on live animal imports. As we have previously reported, agencies can use performance information to make decisions oriented toward improving results.[32] In that same report, we stated that federal managers can use performance information to identify performance problems and look for solutions, develop approaches that improve results, and make other important management decisions, including those that affect future strategies, planning and budgeting, identifying priorities, and allocating resources.

APHIS. APHIS has reported performance information on live animal imports that aligns with the goals it established in its strategic plan for its Veterinary Services program office.[33] Specifically, APHIS measured progress on its performance goal of protecting the United States from the occurrence of adverse animal health events. For example, APHIS reported that in fiscal year 2009 it conducted risk assessments on the animal health status of at least 14 foreign countries that have been denied access to U.S. import markets. In fiscal year 2009, APHIS conducted risk analyses in the European Union for the presence of exotic Newcastle disease, highly pathogenic avian influenza, and classical swine fever—a highly contagious virus that can cause high mortality rates in swine populations. Additionally, APHIS reported that in fiscal year 2009 it did not have any disease outbreaks associated with imports of animals from foreign regions that APHIS has reviewed for animal health status.

CBP. CBP has not reported any performance information on live animal imports. As we previously noted, however, it has agencywide and field operations strategic plans that recognize the agency's role in preventing the importation of zoonotic and animal diseases.[34]

CDC. In general, CDC has not developed comprehensive performance information on live animal imports. However, CDC has reported on mortality rates for one live animal import—nonhuman primates. In its 2008 annual performance report, CDC reported that this mortality rate was less than 1 percent for fiscal years 2005, 2006, 2007, and 2008, down from about 20 percent before 1989. CDC attributed this improvement to its instituting facility inspections and new infection control requirements. In that same report, CDC reported on its performance goal of maintaining low mortality in nonhuman primates imported to the United States for science, exhibition, and educational purposes to, for example, reduce the potential exposure of humans to zoonotic diseases, such as Ebola and tuberculosis.[35]

FWS. FWS reported performance information dealing with live wildlife imports in its 2008 operational plan. In this plan, FWS reported on the number of injurious wildlife interdicted at international ports of entry and land borders (270), number of shipments that contained injurious wildlife (54), the number of wildlife shipments physically inspected (31,000), and the number of interdicted wildlife shipments (4,000). This information supports FWS's performance goal of preventing the unlawful import, export, and interstate commerce of foreign fish, wildlife, and plants in its law enforcement strategic plan for 2006 through 2010.[36]

CONCLUSION

With the growth in emerging zoonotic diseases, as well as the risk of other animal diseases in an increasing global marketplace, federal agencies play an increasingly important role in preventing the introduction of these diseases into the United States. However, as we found, gaps in the statutory and regulatory framework across federal agencies increase the risk that some live animal imports will carry diseases into the United States, as was the case for African rodents carrying monkeypox in 2003. Of the three agencies responsible for regulating live animal imports for disease risks—APHIS, CDC, and FWS—only APHIS comprehensively assesses an animal's disease risk or health status, and APHIS has issued a strategy for expanding its role in overseeing nonagricultural animals. In contrast, CDC and FWS have gaps in their oversight of disease risks from live animal imports. CDC's regulations direct its focus to particular species or diseases, and the agency does not have a process for identifying risks from some emerging diseases that could be imported in live animals. FWS generally does not restrict the entry of imported wildlife that may pose disease risks and does not generally assess the disease risk or health status of these animals. Experts responding to our survey indicated that changes are needed in FWS's statutory authority, its regulations, or both. Recognizing such issues, APHIS, CDC, and FWS have separately proposed additional actions to better protect against disease risks from live imported animals, including actions that may involve pre-import screening.

The four agencies we reviewed have collaborated to meet their responsibilities to some extent. They have recognized the need to work together in their strategic planning, formulated some joint strategies, developed some written procedures for collaboration, leveraged resources in some situations, and shared some data on live animal imports. However, experts responding to our survey and agency officials identified barriers to further collaboration in each of these areas. These barriers—such as different program priorities and unclear roles and responsibilities—are inherent when multiple agencies have related responsibilities. Furthermore, the agencies have largely incompatible data systems, and it appears that some time will pass before these issues are resolved or ACE is able to offer a conduit for data sharing among APHIS, CBP, CDC, and FWS. Because the agencies have not determined which data they will need, it is also unclear whether the data elements in the latest version of ACE will meet interagency needs. While these barriers pose a challenge, the agencies still have a common interest in preventing the introduction of diseases from live animal imports. Recognizing this common interest, the experts responding to our survey, including federal and state officials, reported that increased collaboration through some type of formal entity, such as a workgroup, is needed to help overcome these barriers. Furthermore, the experts and the National Academies of Sciences noted that the absence of a risk assessment system for comprehensively addressing disease risks from live animal imports could result in zoonotic and animal diseases entering the United States.

RECOMMENDATIONS FOR EXECUTIVE ACTION

To better prevent the importation of live animals carrying zoonotic and animal diseases and improve the responsible agencies' collaboration, we recommend that the Secretaries of Agriculture, Health and Human Services, Homeland Security, and the Interior take the following two actions:

- Develop and implement, in coordination with the relevant federal agencies, a strategy for their collaboration in preventing the importation of animals that may be carrying zoonotic and animal diseases into the United States. This strategy should help the agencies
- Identify and resolve differing program priorities so that the agencies can work collaboratively to ensure that live animal imports posing a risk of zoonotic and animal diseases do not enter the United States. Such efforts could include collaborative methods for prevention, such as a comprehensive risk assessment system for live animal imports.
- Lay out individual agency roles and responsibilities for all live animal imports, including how a collaborative effort will be led.
- Identify resources dedicated to live animal imports and leverage these resources to the extent possible to support the agencies' efforts.
- Examine ways to systematically share data on shipments of live animal imports that are regulated by more than one agency until ACE is able to offer data-sharing capabilities to each agency.
- Explore the need for any additional legislative or executive authority to develop and implement this strategy such as the authority to establish a coordinating entity (e.g., an interagency workgroup).

- Jointly determine, in collaboration with CBP, the data elements that APHIS, CDC, and FWS will need ACE to contain, so that the agencies can effectively oversee all live animal imports.

AGENCY COMMENTS AND OUR EVALUATION

We provided a draft of this report to USDA, the Department of Health and Human Services, DHS, and the Department of the Interior for their review and comment. In their written comments, USDA, DHS, and the Department of the Interior generally agreed with our findings and recommendations. The Department of Health and Human Services only provided technical comments, which we included as appropriate. USDA agreed with our recommendations and commented that it appreciates our emphasis on increasing the level of collaboration among federal agencies. USDA also commented that it believes a key component to successfully leveraging the agencies' strengths lies in finding new ways to approach these opportunities and that it therefore supports the formation of an interdepartmental steering committee for the oversight of animal imports as soon as possible. USDA also stated that in collaboration with the committee and other departments, it would seek to determine the need for creating additional authority, clarify the scope of existing authority, and implement current authority more efficiently through expanded memorandums of agreements or other interdepartmental cooperative measures. Furthermore, USDA stated that it would report to us on the components of a successful strategy for addressing our recommendations. USDA's written comments are presented in appendix VIII. DHS also agreed with our recommendations and stated that it would work with the other departments to gauge interest in development of a joint strategic implementation plan. In addition, DHS described its existing collaborative efforts with APHIS, CDC, and FWS, with respect to live animal import processes and agencies' data needs. DHS's written comments are presented in appendix IX, and we incorporated DHS's technical comments as appropriate. The Department of the Interior agreed with our findings and recommendations. In addition, the department provided the following comments:

- While GAO asked experts whether a workgroup should be created to help federal agencies collaborate, GAO did not consider whether an existing body could perform this function. The use of an existing interagency body to serve as a coordinating entity to help federal agencies prevent the importation of animals that may be carrying zoonotic and animal diseases was not mentioned in experts' responses to the first round of our survey, which was the basis for asking this question. Placing a coordinating entity for live animal imports within an existing interagency body may help avoid duplication of effort. If the agencies determine that it is appropriate to place the coordinating entity for live animal imports within an existing interagency body, this response would be consistent with our recommendation.

- The report does not refer to possible confusion that may be caused by multiple agencies having related authorities, and the report could have provided more information on agency outreach to the public. However, as the department noted, the issue of public outreach was not a central question of our review.
- The report should emphasize the National Aquatic Animal Health Plan as a model for federal cooperation with regard to movement of aquatic animal diseases. We believe the report recognizes this plan, stating that it is an example of federal agencies' joint strategies to reduce disease risks from live animal imports, and provided more information on the plan's relevant efforts.

The Department of the Interior's written comments and our responses are presented in appendix X.

Lisa Shames
Director, Natural Resources and Environment

APPENDIX I: OBJECTIVES, SCOPE, AND METHODOLOGY

This report examines the (1) potential gaps in the statutory and regulatory framework governing live animal imports, if any, that may allow the introduction and spread of zoonotic and animal diseases; (2) extent to which the U.S. Department of Agriculture's Animal and Plant Health Inspection Service (APHIS), Department of Homeland Security's Customs and Border Protection (CBP), Department of Health and Human Services' Centers for Disease Control and Prevention, (CDC), and Department of the Interior's Fish and Wildlife Service (FWS) collaborate to meet their responsibilities and face barriers, if any, to collaboration; and (3) the performance information that the responsible agencies have reported on live animal imports. To identify potential gaps in the statutory and regulatory framework, we reviewed relevant statutes, including the Animal Health Protection Act, the Public Health Service Act, the Lacey Act, and the Endangered Species Act of 1973; the agencies' implementing regulations; and agency documents on the procedures employed to regulate the importation of live animals from APHIS, CBP, CDC, and FWS. We interviewed officials from these agencies at agency headquarters and ports of entry. Using information from interviews of agency officials and agency documents, we compared the level of inspection and review used by each of the agencies to regulate the importation of various types of animals, including mammals, birds, fish, and reptiles. In addition, we reviewed scientific studies on zoonotic and animal diseases, including studies by the National Academies of Sciences. We also reviewed APHIS and FWS data on the number, type, and exporting country of all imported animals regulated by these two agencies that entered the United States for fiscal years 2005 through 2009. For the APHIS and FWS data, we analyzed documentation related to the data and worked with agency officials to identify any potential data problems and determined that the data were sufficiently reliable for the purposes of providing background information in this report. We analyzed the APHIS and FWS data to determine the number of animals imported each fiscal year, the countries from which animals are most frequently imported, and the purposes for which animals are most frequently imported. To examine the extent to which the agencies collaborate to meet their responsibilities and face barriers, if any, to collaboration, we reviewed strategic plans, memorandums of understanding, standard operating practices, and other policies and protocols from each of the four agencies. We also reviewed joint strategies developed by interagency working groups, such as the National Invasive Species Council's management plan and the National Aquatic Animal Health Plan. We interviewed agency headquarters officials and agency officials at ports of entry, including airports in Atlanta, Georgia; Baltimore, Maryland; Los Angeles, California; New York, New York; and Washington, D.C.; and the Otay Mesa, California, and San Ysidro, California, land border crossings between California and Mexico, on ongoing and planned efforts for coordination. We obtained documentation on the allocation of staff resources. Finally, we assessed the agencies' collaboration efforts according to practices we identified that can help enhance and sustain collaboration among federal agencies. To help address the first two objectives, we conducted a two-round survey to identify (1) potential gaps in the current statutory and regulatory framework that may allow for the introduction of and spread of zoonotic and animal diseases, (2) how well the responsible federal agencies work together to meet their responsibilities, and

(3) potential barriers to collaboration. The process we followed is based on GAO guidance for identifying experts for panels or other work requiring expertise in a specific area. We identified potential experts on disease risk posed by live animal imports who had primary employment responsibilities related to or dependent on live animal imports, authored peer-reviewed papers, presented at professional conferences, provided testimony on the subject matter to Congress, or were recognized by their peers as experts on live animal imports. We then selected experts from federal and state government, academia, nongovernmental organizations, and industry to obtain a broad spectrum of views. We conducted pretests with several survey recipients prior to distributing both surveys. The goals of the pretests were to ensure that (1) the questions were clear and unambiguous and (2) terminology was used correctly. The first round of the survey consisted of five open-ended questions (questions that solicit additional information) in which experts provided their opinions on gaps in the current statutory and regulatory framework, how well the responsible federal agencies work together to meet their responsibilities, and potential barriers to collaboration. In the first round, we received responses from 33 out of the 39 experts contacted, resulting in a response rate of about 85 percent. We performed a content analysis of the responses to the open-ended questions in order to compile a list of gaps in the statutory and regulatory framework, corrective actions to address those gaps, the effectiveness of federal agencies' collaboration, and barriers to federal agencies' collaboration mentioned by the experts. We used this list to construct the second round of survey questions. These were primarily closed-ended (questions with a set of answers to choose from). We expanded our second round of the survey to include additional experts recommended by those responding to our first round and other experts. Of the 64 experts we contacted, 56 provided responses, resulting in a response rate of about 88 percent in the second round. The first round of the survey was conducted from January through February 2010, and the second round was conducted from April through May 2010. To the extent possible, we followed up with experts to clarify their responses. The questions and aggregated responses are presented in appendix VII. Responses to the survey express only the views of the experts. To examine what performance information the responsible agencies report on live animal imports in their planning and reporting documents, we reviewed strategic plans, operational plans, mission statements, and annual performance plans and reports from APHIS, CBP, CDC, and FWS. Review of these documents allowed us to determine the extent to which these agencies set out performance goals, established measures to assess

performance toward achieving those goals, and reported on the effectiveness of their efforts for activities directly involving live animal imports. We analyzed the extent to which each of the four agencies used performance objectives and measures and reports on the effectiveness of these activities for live animal imports. We conducted this performance audit from August 2009 through October 2010, in accordance with generally accepted government auditing standards. Those standards require that we plan and perform the audit to obtain sufficient, appropriate evidence to provide a reasonable basis for our findings and conclusions based on our audit objectives. We believe that the evidence obtained provides a reasonable basis for our findings and conclusions based on our audit objectives.

APPENDIX II: AGENCIES' PROCESSES FOR OVERSEEING LIVE ANIMAL IMPORTS

This appendix describes the processes that the U.S. Department of Agriculture's Animal and Plant Health Inspection Service, Department of Homeland Security's Customs and Border Protection, Department of Health and Human Services' Centers for Disease Control and Prevention, and Department of the Interior's Fish and Wildlife Service use for processing live animal imports for entry into the United States.

APHIS

APHIS restricts the importation of live animals that it has determined may pose a disease risk to agricultural animals, such as cattle, horses, poultry, sheep, and swine. APHIS has developed import processes that depend on the level of risk associated with either the type of animal or country of export. APHIS has a memorandum of agreement with CBP whereby CBP refers live animal shipments to APHIS port veterinarians for inspection. APHIS port veterinarians visually inspect all applicable live animal shipments and review the import documentation, which may include a declaration of importation, vaccination records, and health certificates from a licensed veterinarian in the country of export. APHIS requires that most imported animals that it regulates be accompanied by a health certificate. A licensed veterinarian in the country of export inspects the animals and then signs the health certificate certifying the health status of the animals and whether U.S. requirements are met. The most common type of certification states that the animals to be imported were inspected and determined to be free of communicable disease. If the animals do not pass inspection, the animals are either quarantined and then reinspected or are refused entry. For example, if cattle from Mexico fail a visual inspection for tick-free status, they are dipped and quarantined for 10 to 14 days and then presented for a second inspection. If ticks are found during the second inspection, the cattle will be rejected, branded as rejected, and sent back to Mexico. For those animals that require quarantine, such as horses, importers are required to reserve space at either an APHIS-managed animal import center or an APHIS-approved private quarantine facility. During the quarantine, the animal undergoes disease testing. Animals that test positive for a regulated disease are refused entry into the United States. APHIS has established processes for specific animals and exporting countries. For example, for imports from Canada and Mexico, APHIS has established streamlined processes, such as eliminating requirements for permits or quarantine for some animals. Additionally, commercial birds— birds that are imported for resale, breeding, or public display—entering the United States through a land border from Canada are not required to have a permit or undergo quarantine, as long as they are accompanied by a veterinary health certificate from a Canadian government veterinarian. Commercial birds not imported from Canada are required to be quarantined and tested for avian influenza. In some instances, APHIS restricts the importation of animals based on risk. For example, APHIS restricts the import of commercial birds from countries with highly pathogenic avian influenza and cattle from countries with foot-and-mouth disease. An example of species-specific regulation can be found with imports of fish susceptible to Spring viremia of carp; such species include the common carp and goldfish. APHIS checks that these imports have the required documents, visually checks the shipments to ensure that they are not leaking or emitting an atypical odor, and assesses the animals' disease status if the shipment is chosen for inspection. APHIS relies on a manual process to account for and track the movement of the live animal imports from CBP to APHIS inspection at the border and to their final destination. According to agency officials, APHIS is developing an automated data system, the Veterinary Services Process Streamlining System, which is expected to replace the existing manual, paper-oriented process and will track live animal imports, exports, interstate movement of animals, and veterinary accreditation. According to APHIS officials, the new system became operational in June 2010 and will be able to track live animal imports in calendar year 2011.

CBP

CBP assists APHIS, CDC, and FWS in enforcing their import regulations, has the primary authority to inspect imports, and seeks to interdict shipments of contraband and the illegal importation of live animals and other products while facilitating the flow of legal trade and travel. If there is a problem with a particular shipment, CBP will levy the appropriate fines and penalties. CBP requires importers to file entry documents that describe the merchandise, quantity, value, and exporting country, among other things, and a Harmonized Tariff Schedule classification, which is a schedule of tariffs associated with individual products. All entry documents must be filed before the imported goods are allowed to be released into U.S. commerce. For faster release, importers or their brokers may provide CBP with pre-arrival notification of an incoming shipment by submitting information on the shipment locally or electronically submitting information on the shipment to either CBP's legacy computer system, the Automated Commercial System, or the Automated Commercial Environment, the agency's replacement system. CBP screens the incoming information through its information systems to verify if the shipment meets the criteria or requires further examination or inspection. According to agency officials, if CBP then determines that further inspection is needed by APHIS, FWS, or CDC, CBP will hold the shipment, provide minimal custodial care, and contact the relevant agency. According to agency officials, CBP holds the shipment until an agency representative of the other government agency is available to inspect and release it. According to agency officials, if an agency representative is unavailable, then CBP denies entry of the shipment.

CDC

CDC restricts the importation of live animals that it has determined pose a risk to public health and bans the importation of certain animals. All live animal imports on which CDC has placed import restrictions are to be visually examined by the inspecting personnel to ensure that the animal has no obvious signs of infectious diseases. Dogs and cats that show signs of infectious diseases are to be examined, tested, or treated by a licensed veterinarian at the owner's expense. According to agency officials, other CDC-regulated animals that show signs of infectious diseases, such as nonhuman primates, are inspected at an import facility. For many of the animal imports restricted by

CDC, the agency requires a permit for importation. Imports that are restricted to these purposes and require a permit include African rodents, civets, live bats,[1] and shipments of more than six turtles with a shell length of less than 4 inches. For nonhuman primates only, CDC requires that persons or facilities importing such animals be registered with CDC. If the shipment has the required documents, it is released to a registered importer. Nonhuman primates are quarantined for 31 days after entry on the importer's premises. No permit is required for the importation of dogs and cats. Generally dogs greater than 3 months of age from countries where rabies is present must have a valid certificate of vaccination against rabies signed by a licensed veterinarian showing that the dog was vaccinated greater than or equal to 30 days prior to import. If the dog is more than 3 months old and does not have a vaccination certificate, the dog may be admitted if the owner agrees to confine the dog until vaccination, vaccinate the dog within 4 days upon arrival at the ports of entry, and then confine the dog for an additional 30 days following vaccination. If the dog is more than 3 months old and has a certificate showing a vaccination done less than 30 days prior to arrival, the dog may be admitted if the owner signs an agreement to confine the dog for the balance of 30 days. If the dog is less than 3 months old, the dog may be admitted if the owner signs an agreement to confine the dog until it is 3 months old, and then have it vaccinated and confined for an additional 30 days. Confinement is defined as restricting the animal to a building or other enclosure, in isolation from other animals and people, except for contact necessary for its care. If the dog is allowed out of the enclosure, the owner must muzzle the dog and use a leash. After agreeing to these conditions, the dog is released and the agreement is forwarded to a CDC quarantine station. The rabies vaccination requirement does not apply to dogs that have been exclusively in a rabies-free area for at least 6 months immediately preceding arrival or since birth. Cats are only required to pass visual inspection.

FWS

FWS has restrictions on the importation of certain wildlife. Specifically, FWS restricts the importation of injurious wildlife and threatened or endangered species and related species for which international trade is regulated under international agreements. According to agency officials, FWS inspectors work with public health officials and other federal inspectors at ports of entry to enforce wildlife regulations and ensure the safety and legality of wild animal imports. According to agency officials, FWS inspectors coordinate with the other agencies to ensure that the requirements for animals that are jointly regulated by FWS and APHIS and/or CDC have been met, such as APHIS prohibitions on hedgehogs that can transmit foot-and-mouth disease or CDC inspection requirements for small turtles. Importers of wildlife shipments generally must provide FWS with a 48-hour notice of the shipment's arrival. Commercial importers of wildlife must be licensed by FWS. According to agency officials, the following processes occur at the port of entry. The shipment is declared at the port of entry, and FWS reviews the accuracy and consistency of the required documents, which depend on species and can include declaration forms, permits, import/export licenses, invoices, and packing lists. Following documentation review, FWS inspectors then decide if a physical inspection is required. Common reasons for inspecting shipments include the type of live animal, exporting country, importer history, intelligence on the shipment, outcome of documentation review, or random selection. If the shipment fails a physical inspection, FWS either seizes the animals with the violations and releases the remainder of the shipment or seizes the entire shipment, based on the type of animal or violation. If the shipment passes physical inspection and has the required documentation, then FWS clears the shipment. If the shipment is not selected for physical inspection and the required documentation is present, then FWS clears the shipment.

APPENDIX III: DATA ON THE NUMBER OF LIVE ANIMALS IMPORTED IN RECENT YEARS

APHIS and FWS provide information on the number of live animal imports, the purpose of the animal import, and the country from which the import has been shipped for recent years. APHIS's Import Tracking System records the number of APHIS-regulated animals imported by fiscal year. FWS's Law Enforcement Management Information System records the number of FWS-regulated animals imported by fiscal year. The APHIS and FWS data systems may overlap because both agencies regulate some of the same species, such as certain fish and birds. CDC does not maintain a database on live animal imports.

APHIS

Table 2 shows the number of APHIS-regulated animals imported for fiscal years 2005 through 2008.

Table 2. Number of Live Animal Imports Regulated by APHIS, Fiscal Years 2005 through 2008

	Fiscal year			
Type of animal	2005	2006	2007	2008
Swine	8,114,546	8,638,151	9,511,180	10,374,424
Fish	0[a]	0[a]	7,754,013	7,537,149
Koi carp	0[a]	0[a]	3,370,220	4,211,454
Poultry	10,412,974	9,396,557	6,312,181	3,769,190
Goldfish	0[a]	0[a]	2,086,047	3,540,739
Cattle	1,506,998	2,374,679	2,291,255	2,494,891
Bison	906	12,025	19,307	27,586
Horses	43,553	37,426	30,202	26,301
Ornamental fish	0[a]	0[a]	498,456	7,254
Other[b]	3,225	7,132	4,215	1,949
Unknown[c]	70,496	20,686	10,426	1,852
Total	20,152,698	20,486,656	31,887,502	31,992,789

Source: APHIS Import Tracking System.

Note: At the time of our review, fiscal year 2008 was the last year for which verified data were available.

[a]As discussed below, the agency began regulating the import of fish in 2006.

[b]Other animals include sheep, goats, elk, deer, moose, caribou, reindeer, llamas, alpacas, pet birds, zoological animals, camels, exotics, and reptiles.

[c]According to APHIS, data in this category could not be identified or verified at the species level.

Prior to fiscal year 2007—when APHIS began recording large numbers of fish imports—APHIS recorded that imports of live swine, poultry, and cattle were about 99 percent of its regulated live animal imports. About 94 percent of these imports came from Canada, with the remainder generally coming from Mexico. These animals were primarily imported for slaughter plants or farms. By fiscal year 2008, imports of fish represented about half of the total number of APHIS live animal imports, with the largest suppliers of these animals, including China, Malaysia, Hong Kong, the United Kingdom, Thailand, and Singapore, primarily importing these fish for commercial purposes. According to agency officials, APHIS reported large numbers of fish beginning in fiscal year 2007 because of a new regulation on the import of fish, which previously were not required to have APHIS permits and thus were not counted by APHIS. In August 2006, APHIS issued regulations requiring importers of species of fish that are susceptible to Spring viremia of carp, a contagious, fatal viral disease, to obtain an APHIS permit prior to importation into the United States.

FWS

Table 3 shows the number of FWS-regulated live wildlife imported from 2005 through 2009. FWS officials attributed the decline of live animal imports in fiscal year 2009 in part to the recession, as well as the increase in FWS user fees, which included new handling fees. In fiscal year 2009, wildlife imports came from a variety of countries and were primarily imported for commercial purposes. For example, Singapore and Thailand were the leading exporters for fish, Haiti and Taiwan for crustaceans, amphibians from Taiwan, mollusks from Indonesia and the Philippines, insects from Costa Rica, reptiles from Vietnam, corals from Indonesia, mammals from Canada and the Netherlands, birds from Senegal, spiders from Ghana, and worms from Canada and France.

Although mammals represent a small percentage of FWS-recorded imports of live wildlife excluding imports of fish—ranging from 0.3 percent in 2005 to 2.5 percent in 2008—they are commonly associated with the spread of zoonotic diseases.

The following describes FWS-regulated imported mammals and their associated disease risks, according to FWS data for fiscal year 2009:

- Bovines, including bison and water buffalo, with 201,561 imported primarily from Canada for commercial purposes. The animal family that includes bovines has been found to harbor 15 zoonotic diseases, including Ebola and Rift Valley fever.
- Mice, rats, and gerbils, with 141,060 imported primarily from the Netherlands for commercial purposes. The animal family that includes these animals has been found to harbor 21 zoonotic diseases.
- Old world monkeys, with 24,106 imported primarily from China for biomedical research. The animal family that includes these animals has been found to harbor 13 zoonotic diseases, including yellow fever and Marburg disease.
- Chinchillas, with 4,302 imported primarily from Canada and the Netherlands for commercial purposes. The animal family that includes chinchillas has been found to harbor 2 zoonotic diseases: rabies and monkeypox.

Table 3. Number of Live Animal Imports Regulated by FWS, Fiscal Years 2005 through 2009

	Fiscal year				
Type of animal[a]	**2005**	**2006**	**2007**	**2008**	**2009**
Crustaceans	11,021,121	12,457,692	12,649,912	10,097,441	9,232,677
Amphibians	5,360,493	5,050,831	4,594,679	4,164,832	3,575,934
Mollusks	1,013,423	1,145,732	1,438,519	1,950,384	1,444,248
Insects	1,037,268	971,078	1,105,246	1,714,148	1,208,392
Reptiles	1,591,606	1,440,749	1,469,399	1,187,679	946,243
Corals	711,747	699,348	980,559	840,657	768,931
Mammals	78,488	115,910	237,767	591,322	289,843
Spiders	215,289	241,627	224,872	203,170	175,505
Worms	1,810,855	839,689	322,656	119,268	162,412
Birds	299,983	225,244	246,710	240,250	159,795
Echinoderms (e.g., starfish, sea urchin)	29,553	48,156	22,626	40,111	133,924
Miscellaneous[b]	2,818,367	2,695,776	2,087,462	2,097,805	1,649,071
Unknown[c]	900	246	116	42	145
Subtotal	**25,989,093**	**25,932,078**	**25,380,523**	**23,247,109**	**19,747,120**
Fish	205,539,504	227,125,679	200,289,950	181,531,235	157,377,941
Total	**231,528,597**	**253,057,757**	**225,670,473**	**204,778,344**	**177,125,061**

Source: FWS's Law Enforcement Management Information System.

Note: This table does not include data for imported animals that were recorded by weight rather than number. FWS recorded some shipments that were not individually counted in fiscal years 2005 through 2009, and those shipments that were measured by weight included the following species: fish, crustaceans, echinoderms, mollusks, miscellaneous, amphibians, insects, annelids, corals, mammals, arachnids, and reptiles.

[a]Animals are grouped by animal class. Animal classes are scientific groupings of animals based on common characteristics.

[b]According to FWS, the agency uses this category for grouping multiple species together or when all that is known is the class.

[c]This category represents imports of multiple nonprotected species.

Appendix IV: Examples of Recent U.S. Animal Disease Outbreaks Causing Animal, Human, and Environmental or Economic Harm

Infectious agent	United States outbreaks	Mode of transmission	Animal and human harm	Environmental or economic harm
Bovine spongiform encephalopathy (mad cow disease)	Three cases of bovine spongiform encephalopathy in cattle have been identified from 2003 through 2006, one of which was caused by an imported cow.	Transmitted to cattle through contaminated feed containing, for example, the spinal cord or brain matter of infected cattle. Transmitted to humans through eating the contaminated meat of infected cattle.	Bovine spongiform encephalopathy is transmitted to humans causing a variant form of Creutzfeldt-Jakob disease. From 2003 through 2007, three fatal variant Creutzfeldt-Jakob cases occurred in two United Kingdom citizens and one Saudi Arabian citizen who were residing in the United States. They were likely exposed to bovine spongiform encephalopathy in their native countries.	An estimated $11 billion in losses in U.S. exports resulted from bovine spongiform encephalopathy-related restrictions in the United States.
Chytridiomycosis	May have been introduced through a shipment to northern California in the late 1950s or early 1960s. Has been linked with serious declines almost everywhere that amphibians are present, including North America.	Caused by an aquatic fungal pathogen, *Batrachochytrium dendrobatidis*(Bd). Bd appears to be spreading through the international amphibian trade, the international pet trade, the bait trade, and inadvertently in produce.	Bd is an emerging infectious disease of amphibians, especially frogs.	Bd is responsible for a large disease-caused loss of biodiversity.

Infectious agent	United States outbreaks	Mode of transmission	Animal and human harm	Environmental or economic harm
Exotic Newcastle disease	An outbreak of the disease occurred in the western United States from September 2002 through September 2003.	Transmitted by infected birds, contaminated people, and contaminated equipment to other birds.	The 2002-through-2003 outbreak resulted in nearly 4.5 million birds destroyed. Humans can be infected with Newcastle virus and infection generally causes conjunctivitis (i.e., pink eye). Most often, those affected are workers in the poultry industry or laboratory technicians who handle the virus.	As a result of the 2002-through-2003 outbreak, over 50 countries imposed some form of trade restriction against United States poultry exports. The outbreak caused an estimated $395 million loss in direct and indirect trade. Federal dollars allocatedto the eradication effort are estimated at $138.9 million.
Highly pathogenic avian influenza	In February 2004, an outbreak of highly pathogenic avian influenza was detected and reported in a flock of 7,000 chickens in south-central Texas. This was the first outbreak of highly pathogenic avian influenza in 20 years. Note: Some strains of highly pathogenic avian influenza do not have the same implication for human health. The highly pathogenic avian influenza strain in the Texas outbreak only affects poultry, not humans.	Transmitted by infected birds.	By mid-2005 in southeast Asia, more than 140 million birds had died or been destroyed. Despite control measures, the disease continues to spread, resulting in animal and human fatalities (more than half of the human cases have been fatal). Many in the scientific community are concerned about a global pandemic of human avian influenza.	By mid-2005 in southeast Asia, losses tothe poultry industry were estimated to be in excess of $10 billion.

(Continued)

Infectious agent	United States outbreaks	Mode of transmission	Animal and human harm	Environmental or economic harm
Viral hemorrhagic septicemia	First outbreak occurred in 1988 and affected marine fish in the Pacific Northwest. Outbreaks of a more virulent strain of viral hemorrhagic septicemia began occurring in United States waters of the Great Lakes in 2006.	Transmission is by infected fish, tissues from infected fish, and water that has contained infected fish. Ballast water is considered the most likely original vector.	Viral hemorrhagic septicemia is known to cause fish mortality, particularly for rainbow trout, turbot, and herring, in short periods of time. APHIS currently lists 28 susceptible species.	Although large numbers of fish loss have been reported, long-term economic loses are unclear. To meet federal and state regulations, aquaculture facilities incur additional testing expenses to ensure their fish are healthy.
West Nile virus	Emerged in 1999 and has been found throughout the continental United States.	Transmitted by mosquitoes and can cause encephalitis in humans.	West Nile virus in the United States has infected 29,766 people, resulting in 1,166 fatalities from 1999 through August 10, 2010.	The estimated economic impact of the disease in the United States from 1999 through 2007 was $400 million.

Source: GAO analysis of literature.

Note: CDC estimates that for every case of zoonotic disease reported to CDC, there are likely hundreds to thousands more cases that go unreported. For CDC to become aware of a zoonotic disease, the following must occur: (1) The infected person has to have contact with an animal and know that it was imported; (2) the person has to become ill enough to go to a doctor and remember to tell the doctor that he was exposed to a certain animal; (3) the doctor has to request a lab test, and if a cause of disease is found, the doctor has to know if it is a reportable disease in his state; (4) the state has to report the findings to CDC in a timely manner so that an investigation can be done to determine the source of the infection.

Appendix V: Overview of Federal Agencies' Disease Risk Screening for Selected Types of Imported Animals

Type of imported animal	Regulating agency[a]	Disease testing at quarantine facility	Assessment by U.S. agency of disease presence in exporting country	Health certificate from exporting country	Visual inspectionat U.S. port of entry for disease
Cattle from Canada or Mexico[b]	APHIS	c	APHIS	APHIS	APHIS
Cattle not from Canada or Mexico	APHIS	APHIS	APHIS	APHIS	APHIS[d]
Canadian horses	APHIS	c	APHIS	APHIS	APHIS
Horses not from Canada	APHIS	APHIS	APHIS	APHIS	APHIS
Domesticated dogs	APHIS CDC	APHIS[e]	APHIS CDC	APHIS[f] CDC[g]	APHIS[e] CDC
Commercial birds not from Canada	APHIS FWS	APHIS	APHIS	APHIS	APHIS
Commercial birds from Canada	APHIS FWS	c	APHIS	APHIS	APHIS
Turtles	APHIS[h] CDC[i] FWS	c	c	c	FWS[i]
Reptiles, not including turtles	FWS	c	c	c	c
Rodents from Africa	CDC FWS	c	CDC[k]	c	FWS[l]
Rodents not from Africa	FWS	c	c	c	c
Amphibians	FWS	c	c	c	c

Source: APHIS, CDC, and FWS regulations and guidance and discussions with agency officials.

Note: FWS does not screen shipments of live animals for disease risk, with the exception of imported salmon. FWS requires that all carriers transporting wild mammals and birds to the United States have a certificate of veterinary medical inspection signed by a veterinarian.

[a]CBP does not develop regulations for how to import an animal, so it is not included in the list of regulating agencies.

[b]Feeder cattle from Mexico, which are cattle imported for the purpose of feeding for a period of time prior to slaughter, are tested for tuberculosis and brucellosis and checked for ticks prior to entry into the United States. Breeding cattle are tested for tuberculosis and brucellosis and checked for ticks. [c]APHIS, FWS, and CDC do not perform this type of screening for this imported animal.

[d]Cattle are visually inspected at the quarantine facility.

[e]APHIS requires that dogs imported to handle livestock must be inspected and quarantined at the ports of entry and tested for tapeworm.

[f]APHIS requires that dogs imported from countries where screwworm is thought to exist have a health certificate from a veterinarian from the exporting country stating that the dog is free from screwworm.

[g]CDC generally requires certification of rabies vaccination for dogs imported from countries identified by CDC as places where rabies is present.

[h]APHIS does not have any regulations in place to assess the disease risk of turtle imports. APHIS prohibits the importation of the following types of turtles: leopard tortoise, African spurred tortoise, and Bell's hingeback tortoise.

[i]CDC does not have any regulations in place to assess the disease risk of turtle imports. CDC restricts the import of turtles with a carapace shell length of 4 inches or less to less than 7; it requires a permit for a shipment of more than six turtles that will be used for science, exhibition, or education.

[j]FWS does not screen all shipments of turtles for disease risk. It requires 48-hour notification of the shipment and shipment declaration forms, which provide a description of the animals in the shipment. FWS visually inspects some live animal shipments (e.g., 18 percent in fiscal year 2008). The purpose of the inspection is to determine whether the animals are on the Lacey Act's list of prohibited injurious animals or are prohibited from entry based on the Endangered Species Act of 1973 and international agreements to regulate threatened or endangered species, such as the Convention on International Trade in Endangered Species of Wild Fauna and Flora—as well as to assess whether the turtles are in compliance with APHIS and CDC regulations.

[in] 2003, CDC restricted the importation of rodents from Africa.

[l]FWS inspects shipments of rodents from Africa to assess whether the rodents are in compliance with CDC regulations.

APPENDIX VI: EXPERTS RESPONDING TO OUR SURVEY ON LIVE ANIMAL IMPORTS

This appendix provides the affiliations of federal and state government, academics, nongovernmental, and industry experts who completed one or both rounds of a two-round survey from January 2010 to May 2010 to identify potential gaps in the current statutory and regulatory framework, how well the responsible federal agencies work together to meet their responsibilities, and appropriate corrective actions.

- Biological Scientist, Centers for Epidemiology and Animal Health, Veterinary Services, U.S. Animal and Plant Health Inspection Service
- Senior Advisor for Science and Policy, U.S. Department of Homeland Security
- State Public Health Veterinarian and Assistant State Epidemiologist, Infectious Disease Epidemiology, Office of Public Health, Louisiana Department of Health and Hospitals
- Director, Veterinary Regulatory Support, Plant Protection and Quarantine, U.S. Animal and Plant Health Inspection Service
- Veterinary Medical Officer, Western Region Import and Export Coordinator, Veterinary Services, U.S. Animal and Plant Health Inspection Service
- Professor, Department of Veterinary Pathology, College of Veterinary Medicine, University of Georgia
- Policy Director, Global Invasive Species Programme
- Director, Science Center, Natural Resources Defense Council
- Virginia M. Ullman Professor, Arizona State University
- Executive Vice President and General Director for Living Institutions, Wildlife Conservation Society
- Director of Regulatory Affairs, Taylor Shellfish Company, Inc.
- Veterinary Medical Officer, National Wildlife Health Center, U.S. Geological Survey
- National Director, Veterinary Medicine, PETCO Animal Supplies, Inc.
- Senior Veterinarian, Los Angeles County Department of Public Health, Veterinary Public Health and Rabies Control Program
- Associate Vice President, Conservation Medicine, Wildlife Trust
- Professor and Director, Southeastern Cooperative Wildlife Disease Study, University of Georgia
- Chief, Division of Management Authority, International Affairs Program, U.S. Fish and Wildlife Service
- Special Agent in Charge, Office of Law Enforcement, U.S. Fish and Wildlife Service

- Professor of Epidemiology, Department of Pathobiological Sciences, School of Veterinary Medicine, University of Wisconsin-Madison
- Branch Chief, Convention on International Trade in Endangered Species Operations, Division of Management Authority, U.S. Fish and Wildlife Service
- Executive Director, Global Initiative for Food Systems Leadership and Professor, School of Public Health and College of Veterinary Medicine, University of Minnesota
- Director, National Center for Import and Export, Veterinary Services, U.S. Animal and Plant Health Inspection Service
- Director of International Conservation, Defenders of Wildlife
- Senior Wildlife Veterinarian and Supervisor, California Department of Fish and Game
- Fish and Wildlife Biologist, Branch of Aquatic Invasive Species, U.S. Fish and Wildlife Service
- Wildlife Health Specialist, Arizona Game and Fish Department
- Professor of International Health and of Medicine, Boston University
- Public Health Veterinarian, National Association of State Public Health Veterinarians
- Associate Professor of Biology, and Director, Program in Sustainable Development and Conservation Biology, Department of Biology, University of Maryland
- Branch Chief, Quarantine and Border Health Services Branch, U.S. Centers for Disease Control and Prevention
- Chief, Branch of Aquatic Invasive Species, U.S. Fish and Wildlife Service
- Professor, School for Global Animal Health, Executive Director, Washington Animal Disease Diagnostic Laboratory, Director, Animal Health Research Center, Washington State University College of Veterinary Medicine
- Professor of Pathology, Western University of Health Sciences College of Veterinary Medicine
- Vice President of Veterinary Services, Chicago Zoological Society
- Branch Chief, Agriculture Production, Office of Health Affairs, U.S. Department of Homeland Security
- Assistant Director, Live Animal Imports, National Center for Import and Export, U.S. Animal and Plant Health Inspection Service
- Chairman, Health and Regulatory Committee, American Horse Council

- Amphibian and Reptile Coordinator, Association of Fish and Wildlife Agencies
- Research Branch Chief, Arizona Game and Fish Department
- Wildlife Veterinary Specialist, Wildlife Disease Laboratory, Michigan Department of Natural Resources and Environment
- Vice President, Government Affairs, Association of Zoos and Aquariums
- Executive Director, Association of American Veterinary Medical Colleges
- Epidemiologist, (formerly) Johns Hopkins Bloomberg School of Public Health, Johns Hopkins University
- Operations Specialist, Delta Air Lines, Inc.
- Manager, Live Animals and Perishables, Special Cargo Standards, International Air Transport Association
- Coordinator, Wildlife Management Division, Arizona Game and Fish Department
- Postdoctoral Research Fellow, Center for Forest Sustainability, School of Forestry and Wildlife Sciences, Department of Biological Sciences, Auburn University
- General Manager, Koppert Biological Systems, Inc.
- Supervisor, Wildlife Health Section, Wildlife Disease Laboratory, Michigan Department of Natural Resources
- Eastern Region Import Export Coordinator, Veterinary Services, U.S. Animal and Plant Health Inspection Service
- Assistant Director Zoonotic, Influenza and Vector Borne Disease Unit, Bureau of Communicable Disease, New York City Department of Health and Mental Hygiene
- Assistant Research Professor, Ecology and Evolutionary Biology, Brown University
- Assistant Director for Field Programs, Global Health Program, Wildlife Conservation Society
- Outreach Coordinator, Fisheries and Habitat Conservation, Branch of Invasive Species, U.S. Fish and Wildlife Service
- State Public Health Veterinarian and Section Manager, Zoonoses and Special Projects Section, Michigan Department of Community Health
- Acting Director Agriculture Policy and Planning, Agriculture Programs and Trade Liaison, Office of Field Operations, U. S. Customs and Border Protection
- Vice President, Conservation and Science, Lincoln Park Zoo

- Director, Planning, Finance, and Strategy Staff, Veterinary Services, U.S. Animal and Plant Health Inspection Service
- Corporate Vice President, Veterinary and Professional Services, Charles River Laboratories, Inc.
- Public Health Veterinarian, Zoonotic and Vector-borne Disease Program, Office of Environmental Health and Safety, Washington State Department of Health

APPENDIX VII: GAO SURVEY QUESTIONS AND RESPONSES

Expert Survey: Live Animal Imports into the United States and the Spread of Animal and Zoonotic Diseases

We conducted a two-round survey to identify (1) potential gaps in the current statutory and regulatory framework that may allow for the introduction of and spread of zoonotic and animal diseases, (2) how well the responsible federal agencies work together to meet their responsibilities, and (3) potential barriers to collaboration.

We identified potential experts on disease risk posed by live animal imports who had primary employment responsibilities related to or dependent on live animal imports, authored peer-reviewed papers, presented at professional conferences, provided testimony on the subject matter to Congress, or were recognized by their peers as experts on live animal imports. We then selected experts from federal and state government, academia, nongovernmental organizations, and industry to obtain a broad spectrum of views.

The first round of the survey consisted of five open-ended questions (questions that solicit additional information) in which experts provided their opinions on gaps in the current statutory and regulatory framework, how well the responsible federal agencies work together to meet their responsibilities, and potential barriers to collaboration. In the first round, we received responses from 33 out of the 39 experts contacted, resulting in a response rate of about 85 percent.

We performed a content analysis of the responses to the open-ended questions in order to compile a list of gaps in the statutory and regulatory framework, corrective actions to address those gaps, the effectiveness of federal agencies' collaboration, and barriers to federal agencies' collaboration mentioned by the experts. We used this list to construct the second round of survey questions. These were primarily closed-ended (questions with a set of answers to choose from).

We expanded our second round of the survey to include additional experts recommended by those responding to our first round and other experts. Of the 64 experts we contacted, 56 provided responses, resulting in a response rate of about 88 percent in the second round.

The first round of the survey was conducted from January through February 2010, and the second round was conducted from April through May 2010. While this appendix displays only the quantitative, closed-ended responses, we also relied on the responses to the qualitative, open-ended questions to inform our findings in this report.

The views expressed by the experts responding to our surveys do not necessarily represent the views of GAO.

Round One Questions

1. What weaknesses or gaps, if any, do you feel exist in the statutory and regulatory framework governing live animal imports with respect to preventing the introduction of zoonotic and animal diseases?
2. What corrective actions should be taken to address these weaknesses or gaps?
3. Federal agencies responsible for live animal imports include Animal and Plant Health Inspection Service (APHIS), Centers for Disease Control and Prevention (CDC), Customs and Border Protection (CBP), and Fish and Wildlife Service (FWS). How effectively (or not) do the federal agencies collaborate to meet their responsibilities?
4. What barriers exist for collaboration among federal agencies?
5. During our site visits with regulatory authorities, we heard about their goal to facilitate efficient cargo and passenger import processing while preventing prohibited animals and animal products to be imported into the United States. What is the best way to ensure that statutes and regulations prevent importation of zoonotic and animal diseases without impeding commerce and passenger travel?
6. If you consulted with others within your agency, firm, or organization when answering the questions, how many others did you consult?

Your Background

7. Please briefly describe your expertise. Include professional credentials, membership and roles in professional associations, titles of publications, congressional testimonies, primary employment responsibilities related to or dependent on live animal imports, etc.

Round Two Questions and Responses

Section 1: Participant Status

1. What is your full name?
2. What is your title?
3. What is the name of your organization?
4. What is your telephone number?
5. What is your e-mail address?
6. Did you complete a survey in round 1 or are you a new participant in Round 2?

- I completed a survey in Round #1 – Skip to question #8
- I am a new participant in Round #2 – Continue to question #7

7. What is your background or expertise related to live animal imports?

Section 2: Animal and Plant Health Inspection Service (APHIS)

8. Based on your knowledge of APHIS's statutory and regulatory framework, do you believe changes ARE or ARE NOT needed to prevent the importation of zoonotic and animals diseases?

Response	Number of responses
Changes are needed	53
Changes are not needed SKIP TO QUESTION #10	2
No response	1

9. How much, if at all, do you support or oppose the following potential changes for APHIS to prevent the importation of zoonotic and animal diseases?

Potential change	Strongly support	Somewhat support	Neither support nor oppose	Somewhat oppose	Strongly oppose	Don't know	No response
A-APHIS resources should be leveraged with FWS to prevent importation of animal diseases.	39	10	0	1	2	2	2
B-APHIS resources should be leveraged with CDC to prevent importation of zoonotic diseases.	37	11	2	0	2	2	2
C-APHIS should have the authority to consider wildlife disease risk as part of its existing risk assessment process.[a]	36	13	3	1	0	2	2

[a]One expert provided two responses, "Strongly support" and "Somewhat support" for question 9C.

Section 3: Centers for Disease Control and Prevention (CDC)

10. Based on your knowledge of CDC's statutory and regulatory framework, do you believe changes ARE or ARE NOT needed to prevent the importation of zoonotic diseases?

Response	Number of responses
Changes are needed	50
Changes are not needed SKIP TO QUESTION #12	5
No response	1

11. How much, if at all, do you support or oppose the following potential changes for CDC to prevent the importation of zoonotic diseases?

Potential change	Strongly support	Somewhat support	Neither support nor oppose	Somewhat oppose	Strongly oppose	Don't know	No response
A-CDC should have the authority to use pre-import screening to mitigate the risk of live animal imports	31	9	4	4	2	1	5
B-CDC should quarantine high-risk animals to allow assessment of the animals' health	25	12	5	6	3	0	5

Section 4: Fish and Wildlife Service (FWS)

12. Based on your knowledge of FWS's statutory and regulatory framework, do you believe changes ARE or ARE NOT needed to prevent the importation of zoonotic and animal diseases?

Response	Number of responses
Changes are needed	52
Changes are not needed SKIP TO QUESTION #14	3
No response	1

13. How much, if at all, do you support or oppose the following potential changes for FWS to prevent this importation of zoonotic and animal diseases?

Potential change	Strongly support	Somewhat support	Neither support nor oppose	Somewhat oppose	Strongly oppose	Don't know	No response
A-FWS should have the authority to use pre-import screening to mitigate the risk of live animal imports	38	6	3	4	0	2	3
B-FWS should have the authority to quarantine live wildlife after import	32	10	3	7	0	1	3
C-FWS should classify species that may be carrying infectious agents as injurious wildlife	25	12	3	9	2	2	3
D-FWS should expedite the process for classifying species as injurious wildlife	31	12	2	3	0	5	3

Section 5: Interagency Collaboration

14. Based on your knowledge of the current statutory and regulatory framework, do you believe a centralized agency should be created to regulate all live animal imports?

Response	Number ofresponses
Yes, a centralized agency should be created	27
No, a centralized agency should not be created SKIP TO QUESTION #16	29
No response	0

15. Within which of the following should a centralized agency be placed?

Response	Number of responses
Animal and Plant Health Inspection Service (APHIS)	17
Customs and Border Protection (CBP)	0
Centers for Disease Control and Prevention (CDC)	2
Fish and Wildlife Service (FWS)	1
A new agency created to regulate live animal imports	8
No response	28

16. How much, if at all, do you support or oppose the creation of a workgroup to help federal agencies collaborate in preventing the importation of zoonotic and animal diseases?

Response	Number of responses
Strongly support	44
Somewhat support	8
Neither support nor oppose	3
Somewhat oppose	0
Strongly oppose	0
Don't know	0
No response	1

17. How important, if at all, is representation from the following entities on such a workgroup?

Entity	Very important	Moderately important	Somewhat important	Slightly important	Not at all important	Don't know	No response
A-Academia	18	20	13	3	2	0	0
B-APHIS	52	4	0	0	0	0	0
C-Aquaculture	22	15	12	7	0	0	0
D-Aquariums	13	16	19	6	1	1	0
E-CDC	49	5	1	0	0	1	0
F-CBP	39	6	8	1	1	1	0
G-FWS	52	4	0	0	0	0	0

(Continued)

Entity	Very important	Moderately important	Somewhat important	Slightly important	Not at all important	Don't know	No response
H-International Air Transport Association	16	16	15	7	0	2	0
I-International Civil Aviation Organization	6	17	14	9	3	7	0
J-Livestock industry	21	15	12	7	1	0	0
K-National Oceanic and Atmospheric Administration	20	12	11	7	3	3	0
L-Nonprofit organizations	8	11	18	13	3	3	0
M-Organizations that use imported live animals for research	21	11	18	4	1	1	0
N-Pet industry	24	14	9	8	0	1	0
O-Port authorities	25	19	7	2	2	1	0
P-Poultry industry	18	17	9	10	1	1	0
Q-State agricultural agencies	27	19	6	2	2	0	0
R-State public health agencies	25	16	10	2	2	1	0
S-State wildlife agencies	27	18	6	2	2	1	0
T-U.S. Geological Survey	22	11	13	3	4	3	0
U-World Organisation for Animal Health	25	17	5	3	5	1	0
V-World Health Organization	15	24	8	3	5	1	0
W-Zoos	18	19	11	7	0	1	0

18. What other entities, if any, should be included on such a workgroup?

Answers included American College of Laboratory Animal Medicine; American Medical Association; American Veterinary Medical Association;

Association of Fish and Wildlife Agencies; Council of State and Territorial Epidemiologists; county departments of public health; Defenders of Wildlife; Food and Agriculture Organization of the United Nations; International Union for the Conservation of Nature; National Association of State Public Health Veterinarians; National Institutes of Health; National Science Foundation; Pet Industry Joint Advisory Council; U.S. Agency for International Development; U.S. Coast Guard, U. S. Department of Health and Human Services Office of Global Health Affairs; U.S. Department of State; The Wildlife Society; Wildlife Disease Association; Wildlife Trust.

19. How important, if at all, are the following activities for a workgroup to help federal agencies collaborate in preventing the importation of zoonotic and animal diseases?

Activity	Very important	Moderately important	Somewhat important	Slightly important	Not at all important	Don't know	No response
A-Define the mission and scope of work related to live animal imports for relevant federal agencies	44	6	2	2	2	0	0
B-Identify gaps in regulations related to live animal imports among relevant federal agencies	50	3	1	1	1	0	0
C-Identify overlaps in regulations related to live animal imports among relevant federal agencies	41	10	3	0	1	1	0
D-Recommend new legislation to prevent the importation of zoonotic and animal diseases	27	16	8	4	0	1	0
E-Develop a coordinated national strategy to better align activities, processes, and resources	52	4	0	0	0	0	0
F-Develop a risk assessment framework to identify animals, diseases, and countries for appropriate action	41	12	2	0	0	1	0
G-Develop a research plan to help relevant federal agencies in assessing disease risks	21	23	8	2	1	1	0
H-Examine methods to maximize inspection resources such as reducing the number of ports of entry	32	17	4	2	1	0	0

(Continued)

Activity	Very important	Moderately important	Somewhat important	Slightly important	Not at all important	Don't know	No response
I-Examine challenges for relevant federal agencies associated with state regulations	27	18	8	3	0	0	0
J-Facilitate training for ports of entry staff	26	19	4	6	1	0	0
K-Develop a plan to leverage existing resources among relevant federal agencies (e.g., sharing quarantine facilities, training field staff, etc.)	40	10	4	2	0	0	0
L-Designate resources to be shared among relevant federal agencies for disease outbreaks	28	20	6	0	2	0	0
M-Develop a plan to ensure that data on all live animal imports is available to relevant federal agencies	39	12	4	0	1	0	0
N-Establish an agreement between relevant federal agencies and international aviation associations to enhance cooperation	20	19	14	2	1	0	0
O-Develop a process for relevant federal agencies to confer with each other when entering into agreements with international	26	13	13	1	1	2	0
P-Develop a plan for relevant federal agencies to collaborate in meeting the obligations of the World Health Organization's International Health Regulations	20	16	15	1	1	3	0
Q-Develop a plan for relevant federal agencies to coordinate counter measures against live animal smuggling	37	10	6	2	0	1	0
R-Develop a plan for identifying and implementing existing Memoranda of Understandings among relevant federal agencies	23	23	6	3	0	1	0
S-Develop public outreach and education programs for those likely to come in contact with imported animals to prevent contracting or spreading diseases	26	14	8	7	0	1	0

20. Based upon your knowledge of interagency collaboration at ports of entry, do you believe communications among the agencies are adequate?

Response	Number of responses
Adequate	3
Inadequate	53
No response	0

21. How important, if at all, are the following activities to improve interagency communications?

Activity	Very important	Moderately important	Somewhat important	Slightly important	Not at all important	Don't know	No response
A-Convene regular risk management meetings	25	14	10	4	1	2	0
B-Integrate outside stakeholders into relevant risk management activities	21	24	4	5	0	2	0
C-Designate a process, including interagency communication, for CBP to hold animals at the port until necessary inspections can be completed by appropriate federal agencies	27	14	8	3	3	1	0
D-Establish compatible data systems containing information for managing, processing, and analyzing imports among relevant federal agencies	41	10	4	1	0	0	0

22. Based upon your knowledge of interagency collaboration at ports of entry, do you believe training among the agencies is adequate or inadequate?

Response	Number of responses
Adequate	8
Inadequate	46
No response	2

23. How important, if at all, are the following activities to improve interagency training?

Activity	Very important	Moderately important	Somewhat important	Slightly important	Not at all important	Don't know	No response
A-Improve cross-training on other federal agencies' regulations	35	9	6	4	0	2	0
B-Improve cross-training on state, regional, and local regulations	27	11	10	4	3	1	0
C-Improve training on zoonotic and animal disease risks	35	11	8	0	1	1	0
D-Improve training on recognition of zoonotic and animal diseases	38	12	2	1	2	1	0
E-Improve training on animal identification	29	15	8	1	1	2	0
F-Create liaison positions among the federal agencies to coordinate training opportunities	23	17	4	7	2	3	0

Section 6: Enforcement of Regulations

24. How important, if at all, are the following enforcement actions to prevent the importation of zoonotic and animal disease

Activity	Very important	Moderately important	Somewhat important	Slightly important	Not at all important	Don't know	No response
A-Provide additional FWS port inspectors	31	12	5	3	1	4	0
B-Increase importer user fees to be specifically designated for enforcement activities	34	4	5	2	6	5	0
C-Identify methods to ensure that animals from banned countries are not routed through another country prior to importation	41	8	1	3	2	1	0
D-Increase penalties for live animal smuggling violations	40	8	3	3	0	2	0
E-Enforce penalties for live animal smuggling violations	42	10	0	1	0	3	0

Section 7: Agency Data Used for Live Animal Imports

25. How important, if at all, is making the following data accessible on the Web?

Data	Very important	Moderately important	Somewhat important	Slightly important	Not at all important	Don't know	No response
A-FWS's Law Enforcement Management Information System	14	18	5	5	2	12	0
B-APHIS's Import Tracking System data	15	16	6	5	3	11	0

Section 8: Other Comments

26. What comments, if any, do you have about the issues discussed in this survey?

27. What other live animal import concerns, if any, do you have that we have not discussed?

Note: We used the responses to questions 26 and 27 to inform our findings in this report.

APPENDIX VIII: COMMENTS FROM THE U.S. DEPARTMENT OF AGRICULTURE

USDA

United States Department of Agriculture

Office of the Secretary
Washington, D.C. 20250

OCT 31 2010

Ms. Lisa Shames, Director
Natural Resources and Environment
United States Government Accountability Office
441 G Street, NW
Washington, DC 20548

Dear Ms. Shames:

The United States Department of Agriculture (USDA) appreciates the opportunity to comment on the GAO draft report, "Live Animal Imports: Agencies Need Better Collaboration to Reduce the Risk of Animal-Related Diseases" (11-09). While the report contains individual Recommendations for the Secretary of Agriculture, we have globally addressed these Recommendations.

First and foremost, USDA agrees with these recommendations. USDA is deeply committed to the protection of American agriculture, as well as to the protection of farmed animal health and welfare, and to maintaining an effective strategy to prevent, contain or eradicate outbreaks of animal diseases. USDA appreciates GAO's emphasis on increasing the level of collaboration among federal agencies with differing types of oversights for animal importations.

As the GAO audit pointed out, USDA, as well as some other federal agencies, currently has limited statutory authorities regarding the importation of animal commodities that are capable of introducing or otherwise acting as vectors for important diseases of animals and/or humans. Moreover, USDA (and many other government entities) is working to find ways to effectively and efficiently carry out our mission priorities in light of constrained funding. Such enforcement considerations would also necessarily apply to any further authorities that may be sought or realized by a Department. USDA believes that a key component to successfully leveraging the different Departments' strengths, while minimizing the individual limitations of each Department, lies in finding new ways to approach these opportunities.

USDA, therefore, would support the formation of an inter-departmental Steering Committee for the oversight of animal importations, whose co-chairs, representing USDA, Departments of Health and Human Services, Homeland Security, and the Interior, would report the Committee's findings and progress directly to their respective

Secretaries. An USDA nominee for this Committee could be determined by November 1, 2010. If the notion of forming such a Committee received support from other government entities, USDA would support convening the Committee as soon as possible. Prior to the first meeting, USDA would provide input for specific agenda items and would work with other entities to create an agenda that focused on the issues of collaboration and focused oversight as highlighted in the GAO audit.

USDA would also work with the other Departments to create a Committee charter with a clear mission statement, Committee goals and objectives, and progress milestones for increasing the effectiveness of animal importation oversights – all of which would be directly responsive to GAO's recommendations.

USDA believes that among other things, such a Committee could examine and discuss the specific statutory authorities currently supporting the processes in USDA and other Departments by which animals are imported to the United States, with the specific goal of identifying areas of overlapping, concurrent, or non-existent jurisdictions. In collaboration with the Committee and other Departments, USDA would also seek to determine the need for creating additional authority; clarify the scope of existing authority; and implement current authority more efficiently through expanded Memoranda of Agreements or other inter-departmental cooperative measures.

As these factors are discussed and refined, the need for streamlining or re-directing existing resources, or to acquire additional resource allocations, would become clearer. With that added clarity, USDA would then formulate a list of action steps which we would submit in a report to GAO. This report from USDA would outline the components of a successful strategy for addressing GAO's recommendations in a timely manner. Once the avenues of increased collaboration have been identified, USDA would also communicate these strategies with its stakeholders for additional inputs.

Sincerely,

Edward Avalos
Under Secretary
Marketing and Regulatory Programs

APPENDIX IX: COMMENTS FROM THE DEPARTMENT OF HOMELAND SECURITY

U.S. Department of Homeland
Washington, DC 20528

Homeland Security

Ms. Lisa Shames
Director, Natural Resources and Environment
U.S. Government Accountability Office
441 G Street, NW
Washington, DC 20548

Dear Ms. Shames:

Subject: Draft Report GAO-11-09, *Live Animal Imports: Agencies Need Better Collaboration to Reduce the Risk of Animal-Related Diseases* (Job Code 361116)

The Department of Homeland Security (DHS) appreciates the opportunity to review and comment on the draft report referenced above. We agree with the intent of the two recommendations.

Recommendation 1: Develop and implement, in coordination with the relevant federal agencies, a strategy for their collaboration in preventing the importation of animals that may be carrying zoonotic and animal diseases from entering the United States. This strategy should help the agencies

- Identify and resolve differing program priorities so that the agencies can work collaboratively to ensure that live animal imports posing a risk of zoonotic and animal diseases do not enter the United States. Such efforts could include collaborative methods for prevention, such as a comprehensive risk assessment system for live animal imports;
- Lay out individual agency roles and responsibilities for all live animal imports, including how a collaborative effort will be led;
- Identify resources dedicated to live animal imports and leverage these resources to the extent possible to support the agencies' efforts;
- Examine ways to systematically share data on shipments of live animal imports that are regulated by more than one agency until ITDS is fully operational; and
- Explore the need for any additional legislative or executive authority to develop and implement this strategy such as the authority to establish a coordinating entity (e.g., an interagency workgroup).

Response: The Department concurs with the intent of GAO's recommendation and we will work with the pertinent organizations within the Departments of Agriculture, Health and Human Services, and Interior to gauge interest in developing a joint strategic implementation plan to address preventing the importation of animals that may be carrying zoonotic and animal diseases from entering the United States.

Of note, currently the U.S. Customs and Border Protection, Office of Field Operations (OFO), Agriculture Programs and Trade Liaison (APTL) collaborates continuously with the U.S. Department of Agriculture (USDA), Animal and Plant Health Inspection Service (APHIS) to facilitate live animal imports. Procedures outlined in USDA's APHIS *Animal Product Manual* in Chapter 2, "Procedures" and Chapter 3 "Live Animal and Related Materials" for Customs and Border Protection Officers (CBPOs) and Customs and Border Protection Agriculture Specialists (CBPASs) to make appropriate agency referrals. These procedures include referral information (Chapter 2) and tables (Chapter 3) to guide CBPASs and CBPOs to the appropriate regulating agency for the clearance of dogs, cats, laboratory mammals, amphibians, reptiles, fish, monkeys, and other nonhuman primates. The referring agencies listed are the Fish and Wildlife Service (FWS), or the Center for Disease Control and Prevention (CDC). Also, CBPASs and CBPOs refer horses, cattle, sheep, goats, swine, and pet birds directly to the APHIS-Veterinary Service (VS) for clearance.

Section 421 (c) of the Homeland Security Act of 2002 (the Act), transferred to the U.S. Department of Homeland Security (DHS) functions of APHIS relating to agricultural import and entry inspections. Article 2 of the Memorandum of Agreement between the DHS and USDA outlines the extent of CBP's role with live animal imports. Article 2 (f) states "Referring all live animals, embryos, semen, and other viable animal products to USDA" and to "Notify APHIS-VS when live animals are present." Additionally CBP, OFO has national bird handling standard operating procedures (SOPs). CBP's bird handling SOPs provide information to the ports of entry (POEs) and includes, as applicable, the CBP Offices of Border Patrol and Air and Marine, and list responsibilities for CBP and APHIS. CBP and APHIS have SOPs along the Southern Border to facilitate the inspection of feeder cattle. CBP and APHIS have guidance for coordinating APHIS-VS and CBP processing of live animal importations arriving from Canada at land border POEs.

Although CBPASs and CBPOs at POEs refer all live animal imports to the appropriate regulating agency, they are not solely dedicated to this particular function. CBPOs and CBPASs facilitate all cargo and commodities for the trade industry into the United States. POEs maintain quarantine rooms, personal protective equipment, cages, and other quarantine materials for all birds encountered from all countries including when the country of origin of the bird is unknown. Seized pet birds are held by CBP and turned over to APHIS-VS.

Recommendation 2: Jointly determine, in collaboration with CBP, the data that APHIS, CDC, and FWS will need ITDS to contain, so that agencies can effectively oversee all live animal imports.

Response: CBP concurs with this recommendation and already has work in progress to fulfill it. The draft report correctly details the creation of the International Trade Data System (ITDS) to streamline data requirements across all agencies. The CBP, Office of International Trade has been working in conjunction with the Animal Plant Health Inspection Service (APHIS), Center for Disease Control (CDC), and Fish and Wildlife Service (FWS) to address data needs for each of these agencies. The CBP, Office of International Trade has already established a mechanism where it collaborates with other government agencies on efforts aimed at addressing their data needs within the Automated Commercial Environment (ACE). The process includes the assignment of an ACE liaison to participating government agencies in order to address their data needs. The data elements are then evaluated, streamlined, and included in the ITDS Standard Data Set (SDS), which serves as a common data dictionary for all government agencies participating in the ACE pilot. CBP, APHIS, FWS, and CDC are all active members within ITDS and have initiated the first steps of data sharing within ACE. The concept of operations plan for the APHIS has already been approved by CBP. The FWS have submitted their concept of operations plan, which is still under legal review by both agencies. Both APHIS and the FWS have had their data needs mapped to the ITDS SDS. The CDC has not yet submitted their concept of operations to CBP. However, CBP has begun preliminary discussions with the CDC involving the integration of their data needs into the SDS.

Sincerely,

Jerald E. Levine
Director
Departmental GAO-OIG Liaison Office

Appendix X: Comments from the Department of the Interior

Note: GAO comments supplementing those in the report text appear at the end of this appendix.

United States Department of the Interior
OFFICE OF THE SECRETARY
Washington, DC 20240

TAKE PRIDE IN AMERICA

Ms. Lisa Shames
Director, Natural Resources and Environment
U.S. Government Accountability Office
441 G Street, N.W.
Washington, D.C. 20548

Dear Ms. Shames:

Thank you for providing the Department of the Interior the opportunity to review and comment on the draft Government Accountability Office Report entitled *LIVE ANIMAL IMPORTS: Agencies Need Better Collaboration to Reduce the Risk of Animal-Related Diseases* (GAO-11-09).

The enclosure contains some general and specific comments. The Department concurs with the major findings and recommendations included in the report.

If you have any questions, or need additional information, contact Kathy Garrity, Fish and Wildlife Service, at (703) 358-2551.

Sincerely,

Thomas L. Strickland
Assistant Secretary for Fish and Wildlife and Parks

Enclosure

Enclosure

Department of the Interior
Comments on the GAO draft report on
Live Animal Imports: Agencies Need Better Collaboration to Reduce the Risk of Animal-Related Diseases (GAO 11-09)

General comments

See comment 1.

No reference has been made in the report to the possible confusion that may be caused by multiple agencies having related authorities. Does the public know where to find data/information on imports and restrictions? Although it was not a central question GAO was asked to review, outreach could have been reviewed / analyzed a little more, since it could play an important role in reducing risks of animal-related diseases.

See comment 2.

Also, no reference is made to any efforts to prevent the introduction of diseases in container water. We recommend adding "Federal, state, and NGO partners should initiate discussions to address potential disease threats posed by container water (e.g. water used to transport ornamental fish or other aquatics)."

See comment 3.

The report should emphasize the National Aquatic Animal Health Plan (NAAHP) as a model for Federal cooperation with regard to movement of aquatic animal diseases. In the future, the NAAHP will be broadened to include amphibians and reptiles.

See comment 4.

Specific comments

"Highlights" Page, 2nd bullet: re: FWS regulation of invasive species. The reference to review of a petition on amphibians fails to explain why this is relevant (i.e., because it is a petition to restrict imports of amphibians (***that carry chytrid fungus.***) Also, this is a reaction to a petition and really does not demonstrate how FWS is being proactive in applying its authority.

See comment 5.

"Highlights" Page: "In contrast, the U.S. Department of Agriculture's..." implies an equality of effort by agencies to prevent the movement of diseases in the live animal import trade, but also implies equality between the three agencies with regard to authority. In reality, USDA-APHIS' authority is much broader than that of the USFWS; therefore, equality cannot be inferred. We recommend the following wording: "USDA's authority is much broader than that of the USFWS with regard to movement of aquatic pathogens, and is focused on agricultural species. The USFWS' authority is focused on native aquatic species in the wild. All agencies should work within their authorities and collaborate to better prevent the movement of aquatic pathogens."

See comment 6.

Page 3, 1st sentence: "More than 1 billion live animals were legally imported into the United States for agriculture, clinical research, education and exhibition, and the aquarium and pet industries." Suggest adding "and other uses" - There are other possible uses that do not need to be mentioned but should at least be acknowledged (e.g., furs).

See comment 7.

Page 4, 2nd bullet: "The Department of the Interior's Fish and Wildlife Service (FWS) administers the prohibition against the import of live animals..." FWS also has the authority to list dead organisms as injurious wildlife, and has done so specifically in the case of salmonids to mitigate the risk of disease transmission, the key element of the GAO report. This omission occurs elsewhere in the report and should be corrected (pages 9 and 20).

See comment 8.

Page 8: We recognize that CBP provides assistance to FWS in enforcing import regulations; however, we believe the responsibilities described are overstated. When a live animal import arrives at a port of entry, CBP does not hold and refer the import to FWS. FWS is routinely notified by the importer/exporter and/or the airline.

See comment 9.

Page 10, 1st full paragraph: "According to the FWS data system, about 177 million live animals – nearly all wildlife – were imported under FWS regulation in fiscal year 2009". The use of the word "nearly" is inaccurate. The FWS regulates all wildlife.

See comment 10.

Page 13, 4th line: it should say "comprehensive science-based" not "comprehensive-based science"?

See comment 11.

Page 21, 2nd line: Bd pathogen (*Batrachochytrium dendrobatidis*) does not cause a fungus, it is a fungus.

See comment 12.

Page 22, middle of 1st paragraph: "FWS is reviewing several proposals to...preventing the spread of invasive species, including:...developing a risk assessment process with scientifically credible procedures; and supporting regulatory and educational approaches." The statement assumes our current procedures are not scientifically valid. Please revise to state: "FWS is reviewing several proposals to...preventing the spread of invasive species, including:...revising its risk assessment process; and supporting improved regulatory and educational approaches."

See comments 13 and 14.

Page 22, 2nd paragraph: "Experts also identified the need for an entity to help the agencies overcome these barriers." The report seems to suggest a new entity is needed to help improve coordination, yet we already have the National Invasive Species Council and Aquatic Nuisance Species Task Force. No mention is made of either of these bodies, or why they could not effectively serve this role. (Also appears on page 32)

See comment 8.

Page 22: Although Agencies Have Collaborated to Meet Common Goals, They Face Barriers to Additional Collaboration – This section states that CBP usually contacts FWS Inspectors to determine whether a particular type of turtle is banned in statute or regulation. This is inaccurate and not a function of CBP. FWS is usually notified by the importer/exporter or the airline.

See comment 15.

Page 24: GAO notes that the principal barrier to collaboration is agencies' failure to take a broader view of the entire importation process. Likewise, GAO statement ".....focusing instead on only those components of the process each agency controls." is not quite accurate, as agency focus is legislatively dictated by authorizations (see comment "Highlights Page" above). We suggest that GAO consider asking agencies to redouble collaborative efforts within their authorities to prevent import and movement of aquatic pathogens.

See comment 16.

Page 30, 1st full paragraph: "While the agencies have worked together...they may not be able to determine whether their funding and staff are sufficient..." This evaluation has occurred as part of the mandate from the Secretary of the Interior for FWS to comprehensively review its statutory authorities, regulations, and processes under the injurious wildlife provisions of the Lacey Act. Recommendations are moving presently through the FWS and DOI approval processes.

See comment 14.

Page 32, last paragraph: GAO asked experts whether a workgroup should be created to help federal agencies collaborate. However, there is no consideration of whether there may be an existing group that could perform this function. Use of an existing body could facilitate collaboration and efficiency by avoiding unnecessary proliferation of groups. The National Invasive Species Council (NISC) was established by Executive Order 13112 (EO) to improve coordination and collaboration among federal agencies and with experts and stakeholders on invasive species issues, including the risk of animal related diseases being introduced by invasive species. The Department of Homeland Security and the Department of Health and Human Services are members of NISC; while the Department of the Interior and the Department of Agriculture are co-chairs of NISC. The EO also established the Invasive Species Advisory Committee (ISAC) which includes nonfederal experts and stakeholders from across the nation. ISAC and NISC may establish subcommittees, workgroups or task teams to consider specific issues; and this has occurred to address a number of issues. The report should state that, in addition to the option of creating a new workgroup, there may be an existing group whose scope could be expanded to play this role.

See comment 17.

Page 55, Appendix V Note at the bottom of the table: indicates that FWS only screens shipments of live animals for disease risk for salmon and CITES listed species only. This is inaccurate. Our regulations also require the trade to provide health certificates for all mammals and birds that are wildlife.

The following are GAO's comments on the Department of the Interior's letter.

GAO Comments

1. In the report, we state that federal agencies face a range of barriers when they attempt to collaborate with other agencies and that these barriers

can confuse and frustrate program customers. In addition, as the Department of the Interior notes, this issue was not part of our objectives.

2. Our report does not attempt to describe all of the pathways by which live animal imports could introduce diseases into the United States. However, we modified the report to include a reference to container water in which aquatic animals are transported as a potential pathway.

3. In the report, we state that the National Aquatic Animal Health Plan is an example of federal agencies' joint strategies to reduce disease risks from live animal imports. We have added language to provide more information on this plan's relevant efforts.

4. We revised the report to reflect this comment by deleting from the highlights page the reference to FWS's review of a petition on amphibians.

5. We added language to the highlights page to clarify that FWS was directed to review statutory authorities and regulations to address existing problems associated with nonnative live animals.

6. We added language to the report to clarify that imported live animals are used for additional purposes.

7. We modified language in the report to clarify that FWS' authority to list organisms as injurious wildlife is not limited to live animals.

8. We modified the report to attribute a description of CBP's processes to CBP officials only.

9. We modified the report to clarify that FWS regulates all wildlife.

10. We did not change the language because it is a quote from the cited National Academies of Sciences report that we attributed.

11. We modified the report to clarify that the Bd pathogen is a fungus.

12. We modified the report to clarify that FWS is revising its risk assessment procedures.

13. The National Invasive Species Council's activities to help federal agencies collaborate are described in the report. We added information on the Invasive Species Advisory Committee, which works closely with the National Invasive Species Council. In addition, we added information on the Aquatic Nuisance Species Task Force.

14. The use of an existing interagency body to serve as a coordinating entity to help federal agencies prevent the importation of animals that may be carrying zoonotic and animal diseases was not mentioned in experts' responses to the first round of our survey, which was the basis for our second round of survey questions. Placing a coordinating entity for live animal imports within an existing interagency body may help in avoiding duplication of effort. We recommended the development and implementation of a strategy to help the

agencies explore the need for any additional legislative or executive authority to develop and implement this strategy, such as the authority to establish a coordinating entity (e.g., an interagency workgroup). If the agencies determine that it is appropriate to place the coordinating entity for live animal imports within an existing interagency body, this response would be consistent with our recommendation.

15. We modified the report to clarify that agencies focus on only those components of the process each agency controls under its statutory authority. As noted in the report, in January 2010, the Secretary of the Interior directed FWS to comprehensively review statutory authorities and regulations.

16. We modified the report to add that an evaluation of the amount of FWS's funding and level of staff for live animal imports has occurred.

17. We modified the report to clarify that FWS requires that all carriers transporting wild mammals and birds to the United States have a certificate of veterinary medical inspection signed by a veterinarian.

End Notes

[1] GAO, Results-Oriented Government: Practices That Can Help Enhance and Sustain Collaboration among Federal Agencies, GAO-06-15 (Washington, D.C.: Oct. 21, 2005).

[2] GAO, Avian Influenza: USDA Has Taken Important Steps to Prepare for Outbreaks, but Better Planning Could Improve Response, GAO-07-652 (Washington, D.C.: June 11, 2007).

[3] Other federal agencies also have specific responsibilities. For example, under the Marine Mammal Protection Act, the Department of Commerce's National Marine Fisheries Service administers prohibitions on the importation of certain marine mammals.

[4] Invasive species may prey upon, displace, or otherwise harm native species. Some invasive species also alter ecosystem processes, transport disease, interfere with crop production, or cause disease in animals or humans.

[5] According to APHIS and FWS officials, the two data systems may overlap because the agencies regulate some of the same species, such as birds and certain fish. As such, the total number of imported animals is not the sum of each agency's total number of reported animals.

[6] GAO, Managing for Results: Barriers to Interagency Coordination, GAO/GGD-00-106 (Washington, D.C.: Mar. 29, 2000).

[7] GAO-06-15.

[8] American Veterinary Medical Association, One Health: A New Professional Imperative (2008).

[9] Exec. Order No. 13,112, 64 Fed. Reg. 6183(Feb. 3, 1999).

[10] National Research Council of the National Academies, Committee on Assessing the Nation's Framework for Addressing Animal Diseases, Animal Health at the Crossroads: Preventing, Detecting, and Diagnosing Animal Diseases (Washington, D.C.: 2005).

[11] Defenders of Wildlife, Broken Screens: The Regulation of Live Animal Imports in the United States (Washington, D.C.: 2007).

[12] B. I. Pavlin, L. M. Schloegel, and P. Daszak, "Risk of Importing Zoonotic Diseases through Wildlife Trade, United States," Emerging Infectious Diseases, vol. 15, no. 11 (November 2009).

[13] U.S. Department of Agriculture, Office of Inspector General, Audit Report: USDA's Controls Over Animal Import Centers, Report No. 33601-11-Ch (Washington, D.C.: August 2010).

[14] U.S. Department of Agriculture, Office of Inspector General, Midwest Region, Audit Report: USDA's Controls Over the Importation and Movement of Live Animals, Report No. 50601-0012-Ch (Washington, D.C.: March 2008).

[15] U.S. Department of Agriculture, Animal and Plant Health Inspection Service, VS2015: A Strategic Look at the Future of APHIS' Veterinary Services, (October 2008).

[16] FWS clarified the number of species listed as injurious under the Lacey Act as at least 231 species, including 100 species of walking catfish, 60 species of flying fox or fruit bats, 28 species of snakehead fish, and 19 species of mongoose.

[17] On March 23, 2010, the House Committee on Natural Resources' Subcommittee on National Parks, Forests and Public Lands and Subcommittee on Insular Affairs, Oceans and Wildlife held a joint hearing, "How to Manage Large Constrictor Snakes And Other Invasive Species."

[18] GAO/GGD-00-106.

[19] The Department of Health and Human Services is currently reviewing public comments on its strategic plan.

[20] GAO-06-15.

[21] GAO-06-15.

[22] National Aquatic Animal Health Task Force, National Aquatic Animal Health Plan (August 2008).

[23] This plan was developed by a task force commissioned by the Joint Subcommittee on Aquaculture, which was authorized by the National Aquaculture Act of 1980. Its mission is to increase the overall effectiveness and productivity of federal aquaculture research, transfer, and assistance programs.

[24] According to the task force, aquatic nuisance species are aquatic and terrestrial organisms, introduced into new habitats throughout the United States and other areas of the world, that produce harmful impacts on aquatic natural resources in these ecosystems and on the human use of these resources.

[25] Pub .L. No. 101-646 104 Stat. 2761.

[26] GAO-06-15.

[27] GAO, National Security: Key Challenges and Solutions to Strengthen Interagency Collaboration, GAO-10-822T (Washington, D.C.: June 9, 2010).

[28] According to the Department of the Interior, such an evaluation has occurred at the direction of the Secretary of the Interior. FWS was directed to comprehensively review its statutory authorities, regulations, and processes under the injurious wildlife provisions of the Lacey Act, and recommendations are moving presently through the FWS and department approval processes.

[29] GAO-06-15.

[30] GAO-06-15.

[31] Section 405 of the Security and Accountability for Every Port Act of 2006 (SAFE Port Act), Pub. L. No. 109-347, 120 Stat. 1884, requires the Secretary of the Treasury to oversee the establishment of a comprehensive information system, and requires a report to be submitted to the Committee on Finance, United States Senate, and Committee on Ways and Means,

House of Representatives, each fiscal year. The most recent report was submitted in September 2009.

[32] GAO, Managing for Results: Enhancing Agency Use of Performance Information for Management Decision Making, GAO-05-927 (Washington, D.C.: September 2005).

[33] APHIS, Veterinary Services Strategic Plan, FY06-FY11.

[34] CBP, Strategic Plan FY2009-2014 (Washington, D.C.: July 2009) and CBP, Field Operations Strategic Plan FY2007-2011 (Washington, D.C.: September 2006).

[35] CDC, FY2008 Centers for Disease Control and Prevention Annual Performance Report.

[36] FWS, Office of Law Enforcement Strategic Plan 2006- 2010 (December 2005).

End Notes for Appendix II

[1] Imported live bats do not have a specific regulation. However, CDC regulates bats as a vector for infectious diseases. CDC defines a vector as an animal that conveys or is capable of conveying infectious agents from a person or animal to another person or animal.

In: Live Animal Imports and Disease
Editors: M. Grayson and P. McLain
ISBN: 978-1-62618-275-2

Chapter 2

USDA'S CONTROLS OVER ANIMAL IMPORT CENTERS*

U.S. Department of Agriculture

DATE: August 13, 2010
TO: Cindy J. Smith
Administrator
Animal and Plant Health Inspection Service
ATTN: Joanne Munno
Deputy Administrator
Marketing and Regulatory Programs Business Services
FROM: Gil H. Harden /s/
Assistant Inspector General for Audit

SUBJECT: USDA's Controls Over Animal Import Centers

This report presents the results of the subject review. Your written response to this official draft is included at the end of this report. Excerpts of your June 29, 2010, response and the Office of Inspector General's position are incorporated in the applicable sections of the report.

Based on your written response, we are accepting your management decision for Recommendations 1, 2, 5, 8, 9, 11 and 12. Please follow your

* This is an edited, reformatted and augmented version of U.S. Department of Agriculture, Office of Inspector General, Publication No. Audit Report 33601-11-Ch, dated August 2010.

agency's internal procedures in forwarding documentation for final actions to the Office of the Chief Financial Officer. Management decision can be reached for Recommendations 3, 4, 6, 7 and 10 once the Animal and Plant Health Inspection Service has provided us with the additional information outlined in the report sections, OIG Position. In accordance with Departmental Regulation 1720-1, please furnish a reply within 60 days, describing the corrective action taken or planned and the timeframes for implementing the recommendations for which management decision has not been reached.

Please note that the regulation requires a management decision to be reached on all recommendations within 6 months from report issuance, and final action to be taken within 1 year of each management decision to prevent being listed in the Department's annual Performance and Accountability Report.

We appreciate the courtesies and cooperation extended to us by members of your staff during this audit.

EXECUTIVE SUMMARY

To protect the health and welfare of our nation's animals, the U.S. Department of Agriculture's (USDA) Animal and Plant Health Inspection Service (APHIS) regulates the importation and quarantine of live animals. In fiscal year (FY) 2008, APHIS required that 165,000 high-risk animals, such as birds from countries affected by Exotic Newcastle Disease, [1] be quarantined at either an APHIS animal import center or a private quarantine facility to ensure that they were not carrying diseases that might spread to the domestic animal population. We initiated this audit to evaluate APHIS' controls over the quarantine and tracking of animals at quarantine facilities, as well as the user fees APHIS charged importers to fund its facilities.

Overall, we concluded that APHIS needs to take steps to improve its controls over the animal import process, especially as it relates to quarantining animals that may be carrying infectious diseases. APHIS established import policies and procedures for import center officials and port staff to follow, while area officials were responsible for providing supervisory oversight of both import center and port operations. APHIS port (i.e., airport) staff monitors the arrival and transport of imported animals to a quarantine facility, where import center officials observe and test those animals for foreign diseases. APHIS import center officials also provide oversight of APHIS-approved private quarantine facilities.

We identified weaknesses in the procedures APHIS used to handle animals destined for a quarantine facility, beginning with the precautions it took when receiving the animals into the country and continuing to the bio-security conditions[2] at the quarantine facilities themselves. APHIS officials did not identify these weaknesses because they did not exercise sufficient oversight to ensure import and quarantine requirements were met. Instead, they relied on the experience and expertise of port staff and import center officials. The weaknesses we identified significantly increased the risk that infected animals could enter the country undetected through quarantine facilities. In two instances, we found that birds infected with Exotic Newcastle Disease and at least one horse infected with Contagious Equine Metritis[3] had entered the country and spread the diseases to other animals.

When animals are imported into the country, they are met by APHIS import center or port staff who review the importers' permits and health certificates. These documents are APHIS' key internal controls for identifying animals that should be placed into a quarantine facility for observation and determining whether certain precautions should be taken. We found problems with these controls for 53 of 131 shipments selected for review. APHIS import center and port staff did not (1) follow permit instructions which required the shipments to be monitored while they were being transferred from ports-of-entry to the quarantine facility, (2) ensure that health certificates included all required information about the animals, or (3) record the correct country of origin on the permit application for some shipments.

APHIS area officials had not performed periodic reviews of port operations. Area officials trusted port staff to ensure compliance with prescribed agency procedures related to the import of animals, including imports from countries that require additional certification, handling, testing, or quarantine. APHIS established these requirements to reduce the risk that animals imported from countries affected by disease would infect our nation's domestic animal population. Thus, it is crucial that port staff adheres to these requirements to prevent the unnecessary importation and subsequent spread of a foreign animal disease. For instance, one of the shipments in our review included birds infected with Exotic Newcastle Disease, which is a highly contagious viral disease that is 100 percent fatal to all species of birds. When those birds came into contact with other birds in quarantine, APHIS had to euthanize more than 9,000 birds.

APHIS port staff had also not always followed the agency's regulations concerning proper sanitation at ports-of-entry. These sanitation procedures included monitoring the cleaning and disinfecting cargo areas and equipment, and collecting debris that may harbor a foreign animal disease. APHIS area officials relied on the port staff's experience and expertise and, therefore, did not periodically review the port's sanitation procedures. At three of the four airports we visited, APHIS port staff did not follow proper sanitation procedures since they did not ensure that aircraft cargo areas and transport equipment were cleaned and disinfected, and non-APHIS personnel were wearing protective clothing. We observed individuals in shorts and sandals handling foreign animals bound for quarantine facilities. Proper sanitation procedures are important to prevent the spread of foreign animal disease beyond the port-of-entry or from physically affecting the individuals handling these animals.

The APHIS animal import centers and agency-approved private quarantine facilities we visited had physical security deficiencies that increased the risk of spreading a foreign animal disease outside the facility. These deficiencies included single-entry rather than self-closing double doors; torn or inadequate screens over windows and doors; individuals who were not showering as they entered and exited facilities; and contractors that were not disinfecting vehicles when they exited facilities. In addition, five of the six private facilities we visited were not adequately accounting for birds brought into quarantine.

We found that APHIS had not developed bio-security procedures for its animal import centers to follow because it relied on the experience and expertise of import center officials to use good judgment. In addition, even though APHIS had written bio-security requirements for private quarantine facilities, it did not identify or require those facilities to correct quarantine violations. We attributed the deficiencies at private quarantine facilities to agency import center officials who, even though they were aware of the violations, did not enforce agency policies. APHIS officials did not correct the import center officials' actions because they did not review import center operations or the centers' oversight of private quarantine facilities. APHIS officials stated that the quarantine deficiencies we noted should have been corrected.

Further, APHIS area officials were not aware of deficiencies at either type of quarantine facility because APHIS did not require them to review, and had not itself reviewed, animal import center operations or their oversight of private quarantine facilities since 2005.

APHIS area officials were not directly overseeing private quarantine facilities for horses that were being imported from countries affected by Contagious Equine Metritis. APHIS had not required its area officials to oversee those facilities because it relied on State agencies to approve and monitor facilities that quarantine horses. In 2007, APHIS officials performed an internal review that noted this lack of oversight and recommended that agency officials review and monitor State activities. In 2009, APHIS officials acknowledged that an imported horse with the disease passed through one of these State-approved private facilities. That horse infected 27 domestic horses and exposed almost 1,000 more to the disease.

Finally, we questioned the methodology APHIS used to calculate the fees it charged importers for agency quarantine services. The agency's current methodology for determining its user fee rates was insufficient to cover operating costs and provide for capital improvements that facilities need to meet basic bio-security requirements. APHIS had established the user fee rate based on a 1995 time study, which is no longer accurate because it significantly understates the time it takes for agency employees to perform quarantine tasks. According to an APHIS official, the time aspect of the user fee rate had not been updated because it was assumed that the tasks and the time to complete them had not changed since 1995. The inadequate methodology contributed, in part, to the agency's budget shortfall because operating expenses at animal import centers exceeded revenues by $1.6 million from FY's 2004 through 2008. The animal import centers also had deferred many maintenance and capital improvement projects that jeopardized the physical security of the quarantine facilities. Overall, we concluded that APHIS needs to improve its oversight of the animal import process to ensure compliance with prescribed agency procedures, especially with respect to animals from countries that require additional certification, handling, testing, or quarantine. In addition, APHIS needs to periodically review and amend its user fee structure to ensure animal import centers have the financial ability to complete maintenance and capital improvement projects related to the physical security of quarantine facilities.

RECOMMENDATION SUMMARY

We recommend that APHIS develop and implement supervisory reviews of its animal import process and bio-security practices at ports-of-entry, animal import centers and APHIS-approved private quarantine facilities. We also recommend that APHIS develop and implement procedures to ensure the safe handling of imported animal shipments at ports-ofentry, and improve bio-security at the three animal import centers and State-approved facilities.

Finally, we recommend that APHIS review its user fee rate calculations to ensure the agency can finance future capital improvements of APHIS quarantine facilities.

Agency Response

In their response dated June 29, 2010, APHIS officials agreed with all the findings and recommendations in this report. We have incorporated portions of the APHIS response, along with our position, in the applicable sections of this report. APHIS' response to the official draft report is included in its entirety at the end of this report.

OIG Position

Based on APHIS' response, we have accepted management decision on Recommendations 1, 2, 5, 8, 9, 11, and 12 in this report. Management decision can be reached for Recommendations 3, 4, 6, 7 and 10 once APHIS has provided us with the additional information outlined in the report sections, OIG Position.

BACKGROUND AND OBJECTIVES

Background

As the agency of the U.S. Department of Agriculture (USDA) responsible for preventing the importation and dissemination of foreign animal diseases, the Animal and Plant Health Inspection Service (APHIS) regulates the importation of live animals based on the authority it is provided in the Animal Health Protection Act. [4] The possibility that a foreign animal with a disease might infect the domestic animal population is a serious concern. In 2007, the Australian government and that country's horse industry lost over $500 million when a single imported horse spread Equine Influenza to its domestic horses. In the same year, the United Kingdom experienced an outbreak of Foot and Mouth Disease that shut down beef exports for more than a year.

In fiscal year (FY) 2008, APHIS monitored the importation of 24 million animals, 165,000 of which–mostly horses and birds–came from 68 high-risk countries where there was concern that an animal disease was present in the population. As part of its responsibility for regulating these imports, APHIS monitors international disease outbreaks and implements import, quarantine, and testing requirements based on the latest data. APHIS amends its list of prohibited countries and animals based on the known disease threat and the exporting country's effectiveness in controlling and eradicating disease. APHIS is also responsible for establishing import policies and procedures for import center officials and port staff to follow, while area officials are responsible for providing supervisory oversight of both import center and port operations. When importers request to bring animals into the United States, APHIS requires that they provide specific information on each shipment and may require them to apply for a permit. Importers must provide information such as the number of animals and the type of species, ports of embarkation and arrival, and the route and mode of travel. APHIS officials at headquarters and import centers use this information to determine if the animals are prohibited from entering the country or if they should be subject to additional import or quarantine requirements, such as a permit or special handling and treatment. If quarantine is required, the animals in question may be held at one of three APHIS animal import centers or at an APHIS-approved private facility.[5, 6] APHIS also requires a secondary quarantine, at a State-approved private facility, for horses imported from countries affected by Contagious Equine Metritis. Importers must obtain a valid health certificate from the country of the animals' origin, signed by that government's veterinary official. APHIS requires that the health certificate include specific statements regarding the health of the animals, such as confirmation that the animals did not come from, or pass through, a known infected area. When animals arrive at a port-of-entry, APHIS port staff review all required import documentation, such as a health certificate and permit, accompanying the shipment. After the animals are offloaded, APHIS port staff examines them and reviews their paperwork. The animals are then transferred to a conveyance and transported to a quarantine facility, under an the official USDA seal, if needed.[7] If port staff identifies problems with the import documentation, the quarantine facility retains the animals until the problem is resolved, or the animals are returned to their country of origin. As a sanitary precaution at the port-of-entry, APHIS port staff monitors the cleaning and disinfecting of the aircraft cargo area, including all crates and equipment used to transport the animals. Collected debris, which can harbor certain animal diseases such as Foot and Mouth Disease, is then incinerated by APHIS import center officials or port staff.

Equipment accompanying an imported animal may be either incinerated or retained until the animals pass quarantine and are released to the owners.

Depending on the type of animal and the known disease threat of the country of origin, quarantine can last between 3 and 60 days. The animals are required to remain in a bio-secured environment until their release.[8] For private quarantine facilities, APHIS has adopted some bio-security components from the Centers for Disease Control and Prevention's bio-safety requirements. These requirements include isolating animals, limiting entry and exit points to facilities, showering when entering and exiting the facility, and controlling pest and vermin (i.e., rodents).[9] During the time animals are in quarantine, APHIS import center officials inspect and monitor them for any signs of disease. They may also treat an animal with a spray to eliminate external parasites and diseases, and perform diagnostic tests that are sent to the National Veterinary Services Laboratories. APHIS issues a release document allowing the animals into the U.S. if testing and observations show that the animals are free of disease. In order to fund its quarantine facilities, APHIS has authority to set and charge importers fees in connection with the animal import process, including fees for processing import permits, monitoring animals under quarantine, testing for disease, and releasing the animals. In FY 2008, APHIS charged importers $4.6 million in import, export, and quarantine-related charges.

Objectives

The objective of the audit was to evaluate APHIS' controls over the quarantine and tracking of animals at animal import centers and private facilities, and the user fees charged by those facilities.

SECTION 1: IMPORT PROCESS AND BIO-SECURITY MEASURES

Finding 1: Agency Import Requirements Not Met

APHIS import center officials and port staff failed to monitor all in-transit shipments, ensure that health certificates were complete, or record the correct country of origin on at least five import permits. APHIS established these requirements to reduce the risk that animals imported from countries affected by disease would infect our nation's domestic animal population. We found that, for 53 of 131 selected imported animal shipments 10 we reviewed, APHIS management had not provided sufficient guidance and oversight of both import center and port operations. It is crucial that APHIS officials ensure field staff adheres to import requirements to prevent the importation and subsequent spread of a foreign animal disease. For instance, one of the shipments in our review included birds infected with Exotic Newcastle Disease.[11] When those birds came into contact with other birds in quarantine, APHIS had to euthanize more than 9,000 birds.

For imported animals, APHIS requires that specific information appear on health certificates issued by foreign countries.[12] For birds, APHIS requires the veterinarians who complete the certificates to certify that they found no evidence of communicable diseases such as Exotic Newcastle Disease or Avian Influenza during their examinations. For horses, APHIS requires the veterinarians to certify that the horses did not come in contact with other horses affected with Contagious Equine Metritis, and that the horses were not from regions affected by the disease. APHIS also requires the name of the country of origin on animal import permits, and that agency import officials monitor all in-transit shipments.[13]

During fiscal year 2008, APHIS prepared or reviewed import documents (i.e., permits, releases, and health certificates) related to over 1,900 shipments of imported animals.[14] Those shipments involved more than 165,000 animals that came from 68 high-risk countries affected by known animal diseases and were required to undergo quarantine before entering the United States. We selected 131 shipments, involving over 80,000 birds and horses, to review. The animals in those shipments were imported from countries affected by one or more foreign diseases. Our examination found that APHIS import center officials and port staff had not followed all established requirements for 53 of the 131 shipments. The details for each deficiency are described in the following sections.

In-Transit Shipments of Birds Not Monitored

APHIS staff at one port-of-entry had not monitored 22 in-transit bird shipments for the presence of disease. When these shipments arrive at the first port-of-entry, APHIS port staff are to observe the animals in their crates for any signs of disease and then ensure the crates are separated from people and other animals until the next available flight. A senior APHIS port-ofentry official stated that, due to long delays of incoming international flights, it made more sense to have Customs and Border Protection (CBP) officials meet those flights since they were already at the airport. Instead of his staff going to the airport, he independently established a verbal agreement with local CBP officials to monitor the incoming flights and report any problems to APHIS area officials.

It is APHIS' responsibility, and no other agency's, to monitor in-transit shipments of imported animals for disease. CBP officials are not trained to perform this function. For instance, one shipment, involving more than 2,400 birds (e.g., finches, parrots, etc.), was unloaded and moved to a cargo storage area where it was reloaded onto another aircraft several hours later. When this shipment arrived at its final port-of-entry for quarantine, the APHIS port official found 14 dead birds and others showed signs of disease. APHIS' tests disclosed that the birds were infected with Exotic Newcastle Disease. We asked APHIS officials about this shipment and the circumstances surrounding the port-of-entry's arrangement with CBP. Those officials stated that they were unaware of the arrangement, and that it was not customary for CBP to assume duties required of APHIS personnel.

Based on the issues related to this shipment, we issued a management alert to APHIS. We also contacted APHIS port staff at all nine ports-of-entry through which in-transit shipments of birds had passed and found that three did not monitor in-transit shipments. APHIS port staff at those three ports stated that they were unaware of any requirement to monitor in-transit shipments. We questioned APHIS officials about the instruction they provided to port staff and to their oversight of port activities. They stated that the import permits they issued for those in-transit shipments required APHIS port staff to monitor those shipments. They also expected APHIS area officials to routinely review port-of-entry operations to ensure program requirements, including permit instructions, were followed. However, APHIS officials explained that they did not require area officials to perform routine reviews of their ports-of-entry. In fact, we found that one area official had not reviewed the operations at one port-of-entry since 2003. Thus, we concluded that APHIS area officials had not adequately monitored their port-of-entry activities.

In response to our management alert, APHIS officials issued an import directive to its port-ofentry staff. The directive, dated November 14, 2008, stated that until further notice, the national office would issue all import permits for animal shipments that pass through a port en route to an APHIS quarantine facility. The directive also stated that permits would only be issued if adequate APHIS port staff was available at a port-of-entry to supervise such shipments. Finally, the directive clarified that this supervision was not to be delegated to CBP personnel or anyone else. On January 5, 2010, an APHIS official informed us that the directive would remain in effect until a new policy memorandum was issued.

Foreign Animal Health Inspection Certificates Were Incomplete

APHIS' import center officials and port staff at two ports-of-entry had not ensured that foreign health certificates were fully completed for 26 shipments–14 horse and 12 bird shipments. Some of the missing information included the following attestation statements:

- The animals showed no sign of disease,
- The animals had not been comingled with infected animals, or
- The animals did not come from an area affected by known diseases.

We also found one certificate written in a foreign language and that port staff had not translated the certificate into English. 15 We and APHIS import center officials and port staff were unable to determine if the health certificates were accurate and complete. Due to these problems, APHIS officials had less assurance that the animals included as part of the shipments in our review were healthy upon arrival to this country.

The foreign health certificate is one of APHIS' key controls to prevent the importation of foreign animal diseases. The certificates are crucial to agency officials because they rely on the attestations of animal health made by veterinarians from foreign governments. We asked APHIS import center officials and port staff about the missing information on the health certificates. They stated that while they usually ensured health certificates were complete for all shipments, they were more concerned with the condition of the animal than information on the document.

We also questioned APHIS officials, including the animal import center directors with supervisory responsibility for ports-of-entry, about missing information on the certificates. An import center director acknowledged that he did not follow through to ensure those certificates were complete and stated that he accepted responsibility for the missing information. Another director stated that he had not reviewed the activities of port staff, including import documents they had obtained for animal shipments. We also found that area officials had not reviewed the activities of port staff, including import documents they had obtained for animal shipments. In a discussion with APHIS officials, they stated that they expected their area officials and import center directors to review port operations and the required import documents, but they had not implemented policies or procedures to require them to do so. We concluded that since APHIS did not require its area officials or import center directors to review port operations, they did not identify that port staff did not ensure that the required import documents were complete.

Incorrect Country of Origin on Permits

APHIS' import center officials at one port-of-entry had inaccurately recorded the animals' country of origin on permits for five shipments.[16] APHIS requires the animal's country of origin on import permits to determine what type of handling or quarantine is needed.[17] We found that the five permits listed the Netherlands as the country of origin. However, we determined that the horses in question originated in three different countries– France, Germany, and Belgium. We questioned import center officials about the inaccuracies on the permits. They stated that they issue permits based on information that importers listed on the permit applications for "port of embarkation" and the supervisor did not review or verify the animal's country of origin until the shipment arrived at the port-of-entry. We found that APHIS import center officials listed the port of embarkation on the permit because they considered it to be the same as the animal's country of origin. This clearly violated agency policy, which requires that the name of the country of origin must be on animal import permits. Even though APHIS' permit policy was not followed, closer supervision should have detected the errors.

It is critical for APHIS officials to determine the animal's country of origin so they can ascertain whether animals being imported are prohibited or restricted. [18] For instance, APHIS allows the import of animals from countries affected by certain animal diseases, such as Highly Pathogenic Avian Influenza[19] and Foot and Mouth Disease, but it imposes additional handling requirements that are critical to ensuring the health of the domestic animal population. The correct country of origin is important to APHIS' determination regarding the type of quarantine, handling, and testing requirements needed to prevent the spread of a foreign animal disease.

Overall, we attributed the deficiencies in this finding primarily to inadequate supervision of port staff. Also, APHIS officials had not performed or required periodic reviews of import centers or ports-of-entry to ensure compliance with prescribed agency procedures related to the import of animals, especially from countries that require additional certification, handling, testing, or quarantine. In addition, APHIS could provide additional guidance and examples of other portof-entry officials' best practices to port staff regarding the review of import documents. For instance, one port official had created a checklist of required import documents, which included the information needed to complete the documents. We noted that this official had collected all required documents and referred errors or omissions to her animal import center director.

Recommendation 1

Notify ports-of-entry that all in-transit shipments of imported animals must be monitored by APHIS port staff, and import permits will only be issued when it can be determined that there is sufficient port staff to properly monitor those shipments.

Agency Response

In their response dated June 29, 2010, APHIS officials stated that they agreed with this recommendation and they believe they are already in compliance. Procedures are in place to ensure that shipments of animals are monitored by APHIS staff.

Animals that transit the United States to a third country must be accompanied by an APHIS permit. These permits include the requirement that APHIS officials monitor such shipments. APHIS issues transit permits only after confirming that port staff is available to monitor the shipment.

OIG Position

We accept APHIS' management decision for this recommendation.

Recommendation 2

Prohibit port staff from delegating their authority to monitor in-transit shipments to Customs and Border Protection officials.

Agency Response

APHIS officials stated in their response dated June 29, 2010, that they agreed with this recommendation and will include this instruction in a guidance document that is under development. This document will be completed and distributed to ports by October 1, 2010.

OIG Position

We accept APHIS' management decision for this recommendation.

Recommendation 3

Establish and implement policies and procedures that require animal import center directors to perform periodic reviews of ports-of-entry operations, including site visits, to ensure compliance with agency requirements.

Agency Response

APHIS' response stated that agency officials agreed with this recommendation and they believe they are already in compliance since processes are in place for reviewing port-ofentry operations. The management oversight of ports-of-entry is the responsibility of the Area Veterinarian in Charge (AVIC). In addition, reviews of port-of-entry operations are also conducted by APHIS management through station reviews, as described in APHIS policy memorandum 515.1, "Guidelines for Veterinary Services Program and Station Reviews." In this process, APHIS management selects field stations including ports to undergo rigorous review by a team of specialists.

OIG Position

We agree that the agency requires the review of ports-of-entry operations. However, the agency does not require those reviews on a specific periodic basis. As noted in this finding, the frequency of port-of-entry reviews did not ensure compliance with import requirements. In order to reach a management decision, APHIS needs to develop policies and procedures, and implementation dates that would ensure port-of-entry operations are reviewed on a specific periodic basis.

Recommendation 4

Establish and implement policies and procedures for area and import center officials to perform periodic reviews of port-of-entry operations.

Agency Response

In their response dated June 29, 2010, APHIS officials stated that they agreed with this recommendation and they believe they are already in compliance since processes are in place for reviewing port-of-entry operations. The management oversight of ports-of-entry is the responsibility of the Area Veterinarian in Charge (AVIC). In addition, reviews of port-ofentry operations are also conducted by APHIS management through station reviews, as described in APHIS policy memorandum 515.1, "Guidelines for Veterinary

Services Program and Station Reviews." In this process, APHIS management selects field stations including ports to undergo rigorous review by a team of specialists.

OIG Position

While we agree that APHIS' station review process may include an assessment of port operations, there is no requirement that a port-of-entry be selected or reviewed periodically. As noted in our position for Recommendation 3, we are concerned that the reviews would not timely identify and correct port-of-entry officials' noncompliance with import requirements. In order to reach management decision, APHIS needs to provide us with a response that describes the policies and procedures, and implementation date, that would ensure port-ofentry operations are reviewed periodically.

Finding 2: Transportation Equipment and Animals Bound for Quarantine not Always Handled Properly

APHIS port staff had not always cleaned and disinfected aircraft cargo areas and transport equipment that carried imported animals bound for quarantine. This occurred because APHIS port staff either did not think cleaning and disinfecting was necessary for flights returning to the country of origin, or trusted the cleaning company to properly complete the task. Further, non-APHIS personnel, such as airline employees and private animal transport handlers, did not wear protective clothing when working in and around these areas. APHIS area officials had not detected these deficiencies because they were not required to visit and review port-of-entry operations. APHIS officials also stated that the agency did not have the authority to require non-APHIS personnel to wear protective clothing when working in aircraft cargo areas and with animal transport equipment. These deficiencies create an environment where animal diseases could be spread beyond airport facilities.

APHIS requires the cleaning and disinfecting of aircraft cargo areas and transport equipment that are contaminated by animals imported from countries affected by diseases such as Exotic Newcastle Disease, Foot and Mouth Disease, and Contagious Equine Metritis. [20] It also requires agency port staff to take additional precautions to prevent the spread of these diseases. [21] These precautions included the wearing of protective clothing such as gloves, coveralls, and masks.

We visited four ports-of-entry, located within the authority of three APHIS area offices, to determine if port staff were properly handling animals imported from countries affected by serious diseases. Our visits uncovered two conditions that increase the risk that foreign disease will enter the country and adversely impact our nation's bovine, equine, or bird populations. Those conditions involved APHIS port staff who did not clean and disinfect aircraft cargo areas and transport equipment, and non-APHIS officials who were not wearing protective gear to prevent the spread of infectious diseases. The following sections describe our observations for each condition.

Aircraft Cargo Areas and Transport Equipment not Cleaned and Disinfected

We observed the conditions and handling of nine animal import shipments at the four ports-ofentry in our review. We noted that the aircraft cargo areas and transport equipment for all nine of the shipments were contaminated with animal waste and debris. Thus, the shipments were required to be cleaned and disinfected by port staff or a private company under the supervision of port staff. 22 However, agency port staff at three of the four airports we visited did not clean and disinfect the cargo areas and equipment for three shipments of imported animals.

The supervisor at one port stated that he does not require cargo areas to be cleaned if an aircraft is returning to the shipment's country of origin. This action is inconsistent with agency requirements and increases the risk that foreign animal disease will enter this country. For instance, a contaminated aircraft may be diverted to another airport due to inclement weather. At the other airport where we found this condition, the supervisor stated that a private company was responsible for cleaning and disinfecting aircraft cargo areas and should have ensured that it met agency requirements. However, he and his staff did not monitor the performance of the private company because the company was compensated to perform the task and he trusted it to properly complete it.

APHIS' area officials are responsible for overseeing port staff and airport operations. However, there is no requirement that they perform periodic visits to ports-of-entry to monitor compliance with agency regulations. One area official stated that the ports under his supervision had not been visited in more than six years. The other area officials we questioned stated that they maintain regular contact with port officials, but had not performed a formal review in years. APHIS officials stated that they expect area officials to perform reviews of ports, but acknowledged that there was no requirement to do so. In our view, APHIS is missing this key internal control and needs to require such reviews.

Airline and Private Company Personnel Wore Improper Clothing When Handling Animal Shipments

We observed during our visits to airports that airline and private animal handling company personnel were wearing shorts, short sleeve shirts, and sandals when entering cargo areas and handling shipping containers. This was in contrast to APHIS port staff who were wearing clothing such as coveralls, gloves, and masks that protected them from contracting contagious diseases, and from transferring those diseases to domestic animals. We were concerned that airline and private company employees could be exposed to contagious diseases, especially after observing them within contaminated cargo areas and handling shipping containers.

In one instance, an airline employee approached several shipping containers of birds imported from a country affected by Exotic Newcastle Disease and attempted to touch a bird. We alerted APHIS port staff who immediately stopped the airline employee and placed a warning sign on the containers. APHIS port staff told us that many airline employees do not understand the danger in handling imported animals, and the risk of contracting a disease or allowing it to enter this country.

We discussed our concerns about this disparity with APHIS officials. They agreed that all individuals who have contact with animals bound for quarantine should wear clothing that protects them from contracting and transferring disease from imported animals. However, they questioned whether they had the authority to require non-APHIS officials to wear protective clothing when handling animals.

The Animal Health Protection Act (the Act), as amended, requires APHIS to regulate the proper handling and quarantine of animals imported from countries with contagious diseases.[23] The Act also provides APHIS with the authority to require the disinfection of individuals who are involved in the importation of an animal, and their clothing. Thus, in our view, APHIS has the authority to require all individuals handling contaminated animal shipments to wear clothing that would prevent the transfer of contagious diseases to domestic animals. APHIS should obtain a legal opinion from the Office of the General Counsel to ensure that it has such authority. If the agency has the authority, it should require all individuals to wear clothing that protects them from obtaining diseases or transferring diseases to domestic animals.

Recommendation 5

Establish and implement procedures for the safe handling of imported animal shipments at ports-of-entry that would reduce the risk of non-APHIS officials being infected or unknowingly spreading a disease to other locations. Obtain advice from the Office of the General Counsel.

Agency Response

On June 29, 2010, APHIS officials responded that they agreed with this recommendation and will consult with OGC regarding the options for implementing procedures for non-APHIS personnel to take additional precautions. APHIS officials also stated that they are analyzing the risks associated with the movement of avian species through transfer airports en route to quarantine, and is expected to issue a report by August 16, 2010. Based on the results of the APHIS analysis and OGC input, APHIS will determine by September 15, 2010, what procedures are needed and how and when to implement these procedures.

OIG Position

We accept APHIS' management decision for this recommendation.

Recommendation 6

Require area offices to periodically review ports-of-entry operations to ensure the consistent cleaning and disinfecting of aircraft cargo areas and transport equipment.

Agency Response

In APHIS' June 29, 2010, response to our report, officials stated that they agreed with this recommendation and they believe they are already in compliance. The station review process, as described in their agency response to Recommendations 3 and 4, includes a review of the cleaning and disinfection procedures at ports-of-entry. Aircraft are cleaned and disinfected under APHIS oversight at all ports-of-entry where live animals are imported by air. Further, companies are subcontracted to perform such services under APHIS' oversight through a cleaning and disinfection compliance agreement.

OIG Position

While we agree that a station review encompasses an assessment of port operations, including the cleaning and disinfecting of aircraft, there is no requirement that a port-of-entry be selected on a specific periodic basis or timeframe. In order to reach a management decision, APHIS needs to provide us with a plan, and the implementation date, to review port-of-entry operations on a specified periodic basis.

Finding 3: Quarantine Facilities had Physical Security and Animal Accountability Deficiencies

Our visits to APHIS animal import centers and agency-approved private quarantine facilities disclosed serious physical security deficiencies. These included inadequate entry and exit doors; inadequate screens over windows and doors; individuals who were not showering as they entered and exited facilities; and contractors that were not disinfecting their vehicles before they drove those vehicles outside the facility. In addition, five of the six private facilities we visited were not adequately accounting for birds brought into quarantine. APHIS import center officials were aware of the violations at private quarantine facilities, but had not enforced agency policies because in their view the violations were minor in nature. APHIS officials disagreed with the import center officials' conclusions. Also, APHIS officials relied on the expertise and experience of import center officials and, therefore, had neither established bio-safety standards nor required area officials to review the quarantine operations at animal import centers. These deficiencies increase the risk that foreign animal diseases will escape quarantine facilities and infect the nation's domestic animal population.

For private quarantine facilities, APHIS established specific requirements related to the physical condition of quarantine facilities, the procedures used by employees to handle and account for animals while in quarantine, and the procedures followed by contractors and employees when entering and exiting quarantine facilities. APHIS established those requirements based on laboratory bio-safety standards issued by the U.S. Department of Health and Human Services' Centers for Disease Control and Prevention. The adherence to these requirements is necessary to prevent animal diseases from being carried outside quarantine facilities by rodents and insects, or on the equipment, clothing, and skin of individuals who handle animals at those sites.

While APHIS established the bio-safety standards for private facilities, APHIS did not formally require animal import center officials to follow those standards. APHIS officials stated that import center officials had adequate expertise and experience in implementing bio-safety standards. APHIS officials did state that agency facilities should be held to the same physical security and animal accountability standards as private quarantine facilities. However, APHIS officials had not established procedures, such as periodic supervisory reviews of quarantine facilities, to ensure bio-safety standards were met.

We visited all three APHIS quarantine facilities and six private facilities to determine if staff had complied with the bio-safety requirements and if they had not complied with those requirements, the potential impact on the domestic animal and bird populations. We found a lack of adherence to physical security and animal accountability requirements, which resulted in an increased risk that foreign diseases could spread beyond quarantine facilities. The following sections describe our observations and conclusions in detail for each deficiency.

Physical Security Deficiencies

We found that none of the six private quarantine facilities we visited had self-closing double doors, as required by APHIS guidelines. In fact, four of the six facilities had single doors that opened directly to the outside. The self-closing double doors are designed, theoretically, to trap a bird between the doors rather than allowing it to escape directly to the outside environment. We also observed that none of the six facilities had double screens on all open windows. These deficiencies made it easier for birds to escape from, or for rodents and insects to enter into, the facilities.

We brought our observations of private bird quarantine facilities to the attention of the two APHIS import center directors responsible for these facilities. One stated that he was aware of the conditions, but did not believe them to be serious or directly related to the spread of disease. The other director stated that he followed the same process as his predecessor, which was to allow some violations of agency requirements because APHIS' facilities could not handle the volume of imported birds. APHIS officials we questioned about our observations disagreed with both of the import center directors. They stated that these were serious violations and that the private quarantine facilities needed to be brought into compliance as soon as possible or removed from the program.

We observed similar conditions at APHIS' quarantine facilities. For instance, one facility that routinely quarantined birds from countries affected by Avian Influenza had no self-closing doors to the outside. Plus, while we were present, an employee left an outside door ajar when she exited the facility. At another facility, screens had holes or did not fully cover doors for 12 of the 14 quarantine barns at the site. The large gaps between the doors and building structure would allow rodents and insects to enter the facility. (See exhibit B for photographs.) The import center director for this facility stated that he was aware of the conditions, but did not have the time to correct them. We questioned the area official responsible for monitoring this facility. She stated that the last review of operations for the facility, which included an onsite inspection of physical security, took place in 2003. In our view, the lack of compliance by import center officials and oversight by area officials has significantly increased the risk that animals or disease could spread outside the facilities.

Another serious physical security problem we observed at all three APHIS quarantine facilities was that agency and non-agency officials were not showering when entering and exiting the sites. APHIS guidelines state that all APHIS officials must either shower as they enter and leave or at least at the time they leave a quarantine area, and all non-agency officials must shower before entering and when leaving the quarantine area. Plus, equipment used on the sites was not being properly disinfected before leaving quarantine facility areas, as required.[24]

At one site, we observed APHIS import center officials entering and exiting the quarantine area with dry hair, which suggested that they had not showered in or out. At another facility, we observed private animal transport handlers exiting the site without showering and changing clothes. At the third facility, we observed construction workers driving in and out of the quarantine complex without showering or disinfecting their vehicles. We were especially concerned about these conditions because construction workers and, in particular, animal transporters have contact with domestic animals from many farms in different locations. In addition, officials from the United Kingdom reported that construction workers were responsible for the spread of Foot and Mouth Disease in their country in 2007. We also noted that two of three quarantine facilities did not have walk-though showers, as required by APHIS guidelines.

We found that personnel at the six private quarantine facilities we visited did not shower when they entered the site. APHIS' guidelines clearly state that personnel are required to shower before entering a quarantine facility. We brought this condition to the attention of the two import center directors responsible for the six private quarantine facilities. They both stated that it was not necessary to shower before entering a facility and they were more concerned about individuals not showering when exiting a facility. However, the APHIS officials we questioned about this condition all stated this was a violation of agency requirements and that import center officials should be enforcing the policy. We believe that APHIS should implement consistent showering requirements for entering and leaving a quarantine area at both the agency's and agency-approved quarantine facilities, and perform periodic supervisory reviews to ensure those requirements are being followed.

Animal Accountability Deficiencies

We found that five of the six private facilities we visited had not counted birds before they entered the quarantine area. APHIS requires this action to ensure that all birds can be accounted for if a disease is detected during the quarantine period. The five facilities only counted birds when a disease was detected, not when they arrived and were placed into quarantine. This procedure is inadequate because the private facilities, as well as APHIS, would not know if a bird had escaped from quarantine.

We noted one instance where APHIS used shipping documents to account for the number of birds in quarantine after a bird tested positive for Exotic Newcastle Disease. In this case, APHIS import center officials required the private facility to euthanize and count all birds that were in quarantine. We were concerned whether this method accurately accounted for all birds that originally entered the private facility. This concern is based on our comparison of the shipping documents to the number of euthanized birds, which disclosed that 65 birds were unaccounted for by the private facility and APHIS. An APHIS import center official stated that those 65 birds listed on the shipping documents must not have been shipped. However, he did not provide any evidence to support his assertion. In our view, since the birds were not counted when they entered the private facility, it is not possible to determine if any diseased birds escaped from quarantine.

We attributed this deficiency, as we did with physical security concerns, to the lack of oversight by agency officials at all levels. We found no evidence that APHIS had reviewed its animal import centers since 2005. In our view, APHIS needs to develop and implement specific procedures for monitoring quarantine facilities, both agency and non-agency, and require that reviews be performed on a regular basis.

Recommendation 7

Develop and implement written operating procedures for APHIS animal import centers to follow that, at a minimum, meet the same standards required of agency approved private quarantine facilities.

Agency Response

In their response dated June 29, 2010, APHIS officials stated that they agreed with this recommendation and will review APHIS regulations, memoranda, and other guidance regarding quarantine facilities for all species to determine if standards are consistent. If differences are uncovered, APHIS will develop a plan to ensure that operations are consistent at all USDA-monitored quarantine facilities. The review and plan will be completed by October 1, 2010.

OIG Position

We agree with APHIS' methodology to develop new bio-safety procedures, but the response did not state when agency officials will implement those procedures. In order to reach a management decision, APHIS needs to provide us with the actual or estimated implementation date of the new procedures.

Recommendation 8

Perform bio-security assessment reviews of APHIS' animal import centers to ensure compliance with agency requirements and implement time-phased action plans to correct deficiencies noted during the reviews.

Agency Response

APHIS officials responded that they agreed with this recommendation and will augment the processes that are already in place for assessing bio-security. Each animal import center has facility-specific protocols that include cleaning and disinfection procedures. These procedures are evaluated during reviews described in the response to Recommendations 3 and 4. APHIS officials work jointly to correct any deficiencies noted in these reviews. To ensure that current processes are consistent and effective, APHIS will review all current policies and procedures and will develop a memorandum that addresses bio-security in the animal import centers and other USDA-approved quarantine facilities. This task will be completed by March 31, 2011, to ensure sufficient time to conduct a complete review and develop clear and consistent policies that can be appropriately implemented.

OIG Position

We accept APHIS' management decision for this recommendation.

Recommendation 9

Instruct animal import center directors to enforce all agency policies related to physical security at private bird quarantine facilities.

Agency Response

On June 29, 2010, APHIS officials responded that they agreed with this recommendation and stated that they will draft a memorandum and checklist for the approval of privately owned commercial and other bird quarantine facilities to be implemented by December 2010, to ensure consistent standards for physical security.

OIG Position

We accept APHIS' management decision for this recommendation.

Recommendation 10

Require area officials to perform periodic supervisory reviews of bio-security operations at animal import centers, and provide a method for APHIS officials to verify that reviews are completed and deficiencies are corrected by field staff.

Agency Response

In their response, APHIS officials agreed with this recommendation and stated that they believe they are already in compliance. They also stated that the station review program, which APHIS management oversees and is described in Memorandum 515.1, includes a review of bio-security operations and cleaning and disinfection procedures. The reports from these reviews identify deficiencies, if any, and a process is in place to ensure deficiencies are corrected. In this process, the AVIC develops a plan of action to be taken and sends a copy to the import center and APHIS regional and headquarters' management. The AVIC is responsible for ensuring that the actions are completed successfully and notifying headquarters when the review is considered closed since processes are in place for reviewing port-of-entry operations.

OIG Position

While we agree that a station review is an important oversight function and may include an assessment of animal import center operations, there is no requirement that a particular animal import center is selected and reviewed within a specific time period. As stated in this finding, APHIS had not reviewed any of the three animal import centers since 2005 to ensure the timely identification and correction of deficiencies. In order to reach a management decision, APHIS needs to provide us with a response that describe the policies and procedures that will be developed, and implementation date, to ensure that animal import centers' bio-security operations are reviewed on a regular basis and deficiencies corrected timely.

Finding 4: Oversight of State-Approved Private Quarantine Facilities Need Improvement

Imported horses infected with Contagious Equine Metritis entered the country through APHIS approved privately owned quarantine facilities. APHIS authorized State agencies to approve facilities, and to visit them after they become operational. However, APHIS had not evaluated the effectiveness of State agencies' oversight efforts. In fact, APHIS officials at the four area offices we visited told us that they had not visited any private facilities since they were approved by State agencies. Some facilities had been approved since 1997. Recently, one horse with the disease entered the country and infected 27 other horses, and exposed almost 1,000 others to the disease. 25 If left unchecked, this disease could have a devastating economic impact on the nation's equine industry. APHIS is responsible for protecting the nation's equine population from diseases such as Contagious Equine Metritis, which is a highly contagious and fast-spreading venereal disease of horses. APHIS considers the disease to be foreign to the United States. APHIS authorized State agencies to approve and monitor privately owned companies to perform quarantine services for horses coming into the United States from countries affected by Contagious Equine Metritis. APHIS required these facilities to quarantine horses coming from affected countries for 30 days.

In 2007, prompted by concerns that horses infected with Contagious Equine Metritis were entering the country, APHIS initiated a review of private companies providing quarantine services. APHIS' review disclosed that veterinarians working at private quarantine facilities were not always following prescribed bio-security measures. As a result, the agency report recommended over 20 corrective actions designed to improve the monitoring of Contagious Equine Metritis by private quarantine facilities. In general, the recommendations included the establishment of minimum standards for approval and oversight of these facilities. One critical recommendation was for APHIS area officials to periodically visit private quarantine facilities. During the initial stage of our audit, we questioned APHIS officials about the status of the recommendations. They stated that, due to other priorities, they had not implemented any of the report's recommendations. In September 2009, APHIS officials informed us that they were in the early phase of implementing some of the recommendations. However, they have not yet decided how to implement all of the recommendations, including some critical ones such as performing site visits to private facilities and reviewing of the procedures used by State agencies to approve facilities. Further, they had no timeframe for implementing the recommendations. In our view, APHIS' recommendations were adequate to correct the problems cited in its report. However, it needs to implement them as quickly as possible to prevent an outbreak of the disease. This is especially important because there have been recurring instances where horses with the disease have entered the country and threatened our nation's equine population. Over the past decade, APHIS has identified 28 horses that tested positive for Contagious Equine Metritis. In addition, since December 2008, the agency has been investigating how an imported horse with the disease was able to enter the country and infect 27 other horses. APHIS reported that another 965 horses in 48 States were also exposed to the disease. This condition increases the risk of an outbreak in this country. In 2007, the Australian government and equine industry lost an estimated $500 million when a single imported horse spread Equine Influenza[26] throughout that country.

Recommendation 11

Develop a time-phased action plan to implement the recommendations in the 2007 Contagious Equine Metritis report relating to the importation and quarantine of horses.

Agency Response

In their response dated June 29, 2010, APHIS officials stated that they agreed with our recommendation and they have completed or are working on several actions to address the recommendations in the 2007 Contagious Equine Metritis (CEM) report. Some of the actions APHIS took included the establishment and training of CEM coordinators in each State approved to receive stallions and mares imported from CEM affected countries. APHIS also provided training, in 2009, to laboratory staff that conduct CEM testing. In addition, APHIS is in the process of revising its regulations for CEM testing of imported animals and expects to publish the interim new rule by December 31, 2010, and will update the relevant APHIS memorandums after the new rule is final. APHIS is also developing a database by which State Veterinarians and APHIS field offices can input laboratory testing data and animal information on imported animals undergoing CEM quarantine and testing in all CEM-approved quarantine facilities. This database is expected to be completed by March 2011.

OIG Position

We accept APHIS' management decision for this recommendation.

SECTION 2: USER FEE RATES FOR QUARANTINE SERVICES

Finding 5: User Fees were Inadequate to Support Quarantine Facility Operations and Upgrades

APHIS' user fee revenues, generated from quarantine services, were approximately $1.6 million less than the expenses of animal import centers for the period from FY 2004 through 2008. We attributed this shortfall to an outdated user fee rate that did not sufficiently account for the time it actually took APHIS employees to complete tasks related to quarantine services. According to an APHIS official, the time aspect of the user fee rate had not been updated because it was assumed that the tasks and the time to complete them had not changed. Consequently, APHIS' animal import centers did not have the financial ability to complete many maintenance and capital improvement projects related to the physical security of quarantine facilities. This increases the risk that foreign diseases could escape and negatively impact the domestic animal population. Congress, in granting APHIS the authority to charge user fees, expected the agency to recover, to the fullest extent possible, all operating costs and costs for capital improvement projects needed to maintain animal import centers' buildings and related quarantine services. However, we found that user fee revenue was insufficient to cover the maintenance and capital improvement projects needed at animal import centers. For instance, in FY 2008, APHIS collected about $4.6 million in user fee revenues, but incurred operating expenses of nearly $4.7 million. This did not include costs for capital improvement projects for the facilities, one of which was almost 30 years old and in need of repairs. In fact, we noted that there was a shortfall for each of the last 2 years comprising the period of our review. Thus, we analyzed APHIS' user fee rate structure to determine the reason for the shortfall. Our analysis identified one variable in the rate structure, the time aspect related to some tasks, which appeared to be too low. When we questioned APHIS officials about the time factor used in the rate, they informed us that it was based on a time-study performed in 1995. The study evaluated the time APHIS employees took to complete 116 tasks involving the arrival, inspection, testing, monitoring, and release of animals from quarantine. To determine if the study was still valid, we asked the animal import center directors to estimate the time it currently takes to complete the 116 tasks listed in the study. Based on their responses, we determined that there were increases in completion time for 97 of the 116 tasks. The time to complete some tasks increased substantially. For instance, the daily inspection of birds (over the entire quarantine period of 30 days) took 6.25 hours to complete in 1995, while that same task had increased to 15 hours in 2008. Similarly, the time to complete all quarantine activities related to birds and poultry at one import center increased from 1.5 hours in 1995 to 4.25 hours in 2008, an increase of 164 percent. According to the director of that facility, the 2003 Avian Influenza outbreak in Asia increased the level of inspection and monitoring that was needed to ensure that birds with that disease did not enter the nation and infect the domestic population. The director also stated that the time to monitor horses from countries with Foot and Mouth Disease has increased significantly. APHIS reviews its fee structure biennially, but has never adjusted the time variable of the rate. The APHIS official responsible for the fee structure stated that she never thought about performing another time-study because she thought that the length of time to complete quarantine activities had not changed since 1995. In our view, the time factor is critical and should be evaluated by APHIS. This factor, when multiplied by employee labor costs, is critical to determining the user fee revenue necessary to cover the agency's operating costs and fund capital improvement projects.

The agency especially needs to provide funds for capital improvement projects. As noted in Finding 3, we observed many violations of bio-security requirements. We attribute some of those violations to a lack of funding to make repairs or to improve the facilities. For instance, import center officials at one of the quarantine facilities informed us that they did not have funds available for needed maintenance and capital improvement. One of those officials also stated that funds were so low that he had to climb onto the facility's roof to repair a broken exhaust motor. At another site, we observed that the walk through showers in the quarantine barns had not been used recently. These walk-through showers are a critical feature for preventing the spread of animal diseases. An APHIS area official confirmed that the showers had not worked for some time, and stated that there were no funds to make the repairs. APHIS had recently obtained an independent assessment of this nearly 30 year old facility. The assessment report concluded that the facility was in poor condition and needed over $3 million in repairs to fix deferred maintenance items. The contractor who performed the review recommended that the agency set aside a portion of its user fee revenues to fund long-term maintenance and capital improvement projects. In 2008, APHIS published new rates for fiscal years 2009 through 2013 that increased user fees by over 37 percent. However, those rates were based on the 1995 time study. In our view, APHIS needs to revise its current user fee rate structure to adequately provide sufficient funds to properly operate the quarantine facilities and for necessary upgrades. We discussed this issue with APHIS officials, who agreed that the current user fee rate structure was outdated and incomplete and needed to be revised to meet the financial needs of quarantine facilities. Although APHIS changed the methodology to reflect the total costs that need to be recovered, that methodology was still based on the 1995 time study.

Recommendation 12

Revise the user fee rate structure by identifying the funds needed to adequately support quarantine facility operations and upgrades, and at a minimum, update the study for the time it takes to complete all quarantine tasks. Establish procedures to periodically update that study to account for time and cost changes.

Agency Response

In their response, dated June 29, 2010, APHIS officials stated that they agreed with this recommendation. They also stated that they have and will take action to review and evaluate their user fee structure. APHIS officials have completed an internal review of program costs and estimated volumes to determine where the fees need to be increased in order to have full cost recovery. APHIS officials visited the New York Animal Import Center in December 2009, and the Miami Animal Import Center in January 2010, and performed time studies and collected time survey data to use in the next user fee quarantine rate calculations. In addition, APHIS officials plan to perform an in-depth review of all costs to ensure the user fee rates will adequately support the facility operations and anticipated upgrades. APHIS' Financial Management Division staff will work closely with animal import center program management to devise and propose a new user fee schedule and write a rule work plan by October 29, 2010, to take effect during fiscal year 2013. In the interim, beginning in fiscal year 2011, APHIS will establish accounting codes for individual ports so that costs can be better tracked.

OIG Position

We accept APHIS' management decision for this recommendation.

SCOPE AND METHODOLOGY

We performed our audit at the APHIS national office, two regional offices, five area offices, and three animal import centers and associated ports-of-entry. We visited APHIS' three animal import centers in Los Angeles, California; [27] Miami, Florida; and Newburgh, New York. We judgmentally selected and visited 8 of the 16 APHIS-approved private quarantines.[28] (See exhibit A.) We did not visit any of the APHIS-approved home quarantine locations since, at the animal import centers we visited, the controls were in place and functioning as intended. The period of our audit was fiscal years (FY) 2008 and 2009 for import and quarantine operations. At APHIS' national office, we reviewed and analyzed animal import data from the ePermits system and the Import Tracking System (ITS).[29] Both systems process and issue a variety of documents (i.e., permits), including those for animals requiring quarantine, but only ITS records the type, purpose, and number of animals released from quarantine. Based on the data agency officials provided, from a total of over 24 million animals imported to the United States during fiscal year 2008, APHIS issued over 1,900 import permits for more than 165,000 animals requiring quarantine.[30] A majority of the animals imported to the United States did not require quarantine, and of those that were quarantined, only certain animals from high-risk countries need a permit. In prior audits, we identified errors and omissions in both the ePermits[31] and ITS databases.[32] Therefore, we did not rely upon the totals APHIS provided from either system. APHIS officials stated that they will focus their limited information technology resources on implementing a new import module in their Veterinary Services Process Streamlining system. Based on the ePermits and ITS data available to us, we judgmentally selected 131 files for review: 30 files from over 1,800 electronic permits, 42 files from over 4,500 release documents, and 59 out of 99 manually-prepared permits. These files covered import activity for quarantined animal shipments for all three animal import centers and seven private bird and two private horse quarantine facilities. We reviewed APHIS' user fee structure and the procedures to charge, collect, and deposit those fees to the U.S. Treasury. During FY 2008, APHIS collected $23.5 million in user fees, $4.6 million of which comprised import, export, and quarantine-related charges. We also analyzed the revenue and expenditures specifically for animal import centers from FY 2004 through FY 2008. To accomplish our audit objectives we:

- Reviewed laws, regulations, policies, procedures, and memoranda pertaining to the importation and quarantine of live animals;
- Interviewed APHIS national, regional (eastern and western), and area officials to determine their oversight of import center and port operations. We also interviewed APHIS officials at the animal import centers and ports-of-entry we visited;
- Analyzed the information technology systems (ePermits and ITS) used to prepare, issue, and record import data for quarantined animals to identify trends and select files for review. We analyzed the Investigative and Enforcement Services Division's opened and closed cases for import or quarantine violations. We also analyzed the Marketing and Regulatory Business Services' Financial Management Division's user fee structure and collection procedures;
- Evaluated oversight of animal import center operations. We analyzed APHIS' regional station/port reviews performed of area offices, animal import centers, and ports-of-entry. We analyzed APHIS area offices' oversight of animal import centers, ports-of-entry, and quarantine facilities including State-approved private facilities that quarantine imported horses for Contagious Equine Metritis;
- Observed the arrival of nine animal shipments at four airports. We observed APHIS and non-APHIS officials' handling and processing of animals at the airports, transporting of animals to an APHIS or an APHIS-approved private quarantine facility, placement and testing of animals in quarantine, and final release. We analyzed the documents collected by import center and port-of-entry officials to ensure all import requirements were met. We also analyzed controls over official USDA seals and forms at both the animal import centers and ports-of entry;
- Analyzed the adequacy of APHIS' bio-security requirements implemented at animal import centers, ports-of-entry, and APHIS-approved private quarantines; and

- Observed operations and interviewed owners and managers to determine if they followed APHIS' procedures for inventory control and bio-security.

We performed our audit fieldwork from July 2008 through January 2010. We conducted this performance audit in accordance with generally accepted government auditing standards. Those standards require that we plan and perform the audit to obtain sufficient, appropriate evidence to provide a reasonable basis for our findings and conclusions based on our audit objectives. We believe that the evidence obtained provides a reasonable basis for our findings and conclusions based on our audit objectives.

ABBREVIATIONS

APHIS	Animal and Plant Health Inspection Service
AVIC	Area Veterinarian in Charge
CBP	Customs and Border Protection (U.S. Department of Homeland Security)
CEM	Contagious Equine Metritis
CFR	Code of Federal Regulations
FY	Fiscal Year
ITS	Import Tracking System
USDA	United States Department of Agriculture

EXHIBIT A: LOCATIONS REVIEWED

Name	Location
APHIS Headquarters	Riverdale, Maryland
APHIS Eastern Regional Office	Raleigh, North Carolina
APHIS Western Regional Office	Fort Collins, Colorado
APHIS Area Offices	Albany, New York; Gainesville, Florida; Sacramento, California; Conyers, Georgia (near Atlanta); and Richmond, Virginia
APHIS Operated Quarantine Facilities	Miami, Florida; Newburgh, New York; and San Ysidro, California
6 Private Bird Quarantines	5 in Los Angeles, California; and 1 in Miami, Florida
2 Private Horse Quarantines	Los Angeles, California
States with Approved Private Horse Quarantines for Contagious Equine Metritis	Florida and Virginia

The table above lists the locations reviewed during this audit.

EXHIBIT B: PHOTOGRAPHS OF ANIMAL IMPORT CENTER DEFICIENCIES

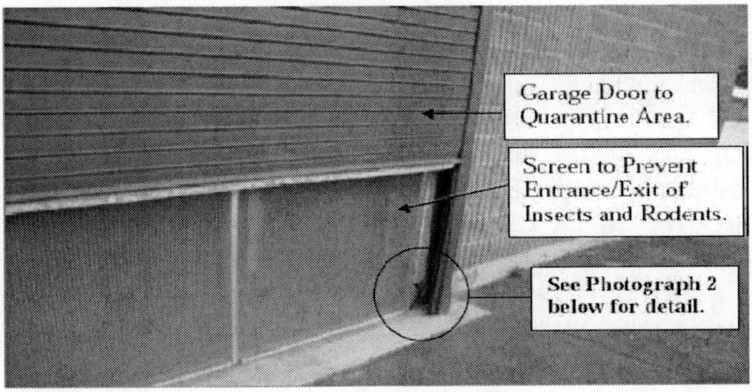

Photograph No. 1, exterior of quarantine barn and garage door partially open with a screen covering the opening.

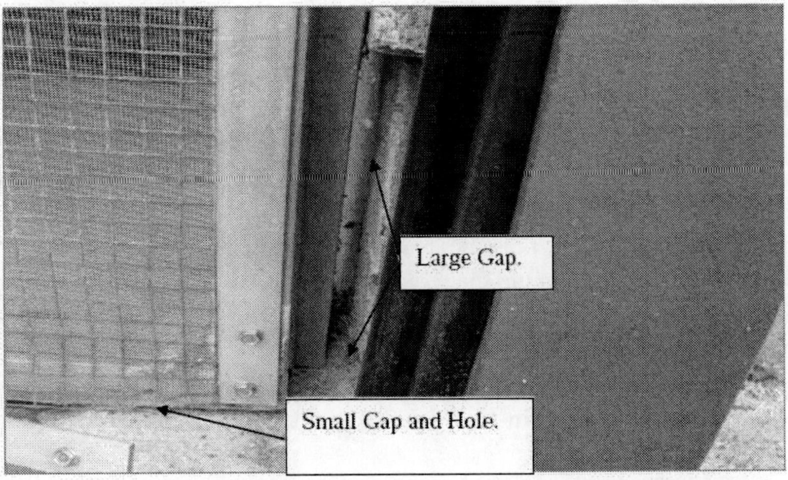

Photograph No. 2, a closeup of Photograph No. 1 showing the gap between the screen and barn wall and a hole in the screen.

AGENCY'S RESPONSE

USDA'S APHIS Response to Audit Report

MEMORANDUM
June 29, 2010

United States Department of Agriculture
Animal and Plant Health Inspection Service

TO: Gil H. Harden
Assistant Inspector General for Audit
FROM: Cindy J. Smith /s/ Administrator

SUBJECT: APHIS Response and Request for Management Decisions, on OIG Report, "USDA's Controls Over Animal Import Centers" (33601-11-CH)

We have reviewed the above captioned audit report and offer the comments detailed below. We have addressed each recommendation and set forth the completed and/or planned corrective actions, as necessary, and the timeframes for their implementation.

Recommendation 1: Notify ports-of-entry that all in-transit shipments of imported animals must be monitored by APHIS port staff, and import permits will only be issued when it can be determined that there is sufficient port staff to properly monitor those shipments.

APHIS Response: APHIS agrees with the recommendation and believes we are already in compliance. Procedures are in place to ensure that shipments of animals are monitored by APHIS staff. Animals that transit the United States to a third country must be accompanied by a Veterinary Services (VS) permit. These permit include the requirement that VS monitor such shipments. VS issues transit permits only after confirming that port staff is available to monitor the shipment.

Recommendation 2: Prohibit port staff from delegating their authority to monitor in-transit shipments to Customs and Border Protection officials.

APHIS Response: APHIS agrees with this recommendation and will include this instruction in a guidance document (VS Memorandum) that is under development. This document will be completed and distributed to ports by October 1, 2010.

Recommendation 3: Establish and implement policies and procedures that require animal import center directors to perform periodic reviews of ports-ofentry operations, including site visits, to ensure compliance with agency requirements.

Recommendation 4: Establish and implement policies and procedures for area and import center officials to perform periodic reviews of port-of-entry operations.

APHIS Response to 3 and 4: APHIS agrees with this recommendation and believes we are already in compliance. Processes are in place for reviewing portof-entry operations. First, VS Area Veterinarians in Charge (AVICs) are responsible for oversight of the ports-of-entry that are located in their areas. As part of this oversight, the AVIC ensures that ports comply with agency requirements. Second, VS management conducts reviews of port operations through its station review program. In this process, VS management selects field stations, including ports, to undergo a rigorous review by a team of specialists. Details on conducting station reviews are set forth in VS Memorandum 515.1, "Guidelines for Veterinary Services Program and Station Reviews," and an accompanying station review guide.

Recommendation 5: Establish and implement procedures for the safe handling of imported animal shipments at ports-of-entry that would reduce the risk of non-APHIS officials being infected or unknowingly spreading a disease to other locations. Obtain advice from the Office of General Counsel.

APHIS Response: APHIS agrees with this recommendation. VS will consult with the Office of General Counsel (OGC) regarding options for implementing additional precautionary procedures for non APHIS personnel. In particular, VS is analyzing the risks associated with the movement of avian species through transfer airports en route to quarantine. The analysis (and an accompanying report) will be completed by August 16, 2010. Based on this report and input from OGC, VS will determine what procedures are needed by September 15, 2010. By November 1, we will develop a plan and timetable for implementation of new or revised procedures.

The OIG audit report cited a specific case involving an airline employee's handling of a container of birds that originated from a country affected by Newcastle disease. All birds imported from such countries must be certified by the exporting country as healthy and as not having been exposed to Newcastle disease within the previous 60 days. Therefore, the potential for human exposure to avian diseases is minimal.

Recommendation 6: Require area offices to periodically review ports-of-entry operations to ensure the consistent application of cleaning and disinfecting aircraft cargo areas and transport equipment.

APHIS Response: APHIS agrees with this recommendation and believes we are already in compliance. The review processes described in the response to recommendations 3 and 4 include a review of cleaning and disinfection procedures at ports. Aircraft are cleaned and disinfected under VS oversight at all ports-ofentry where live animals are imported by air. Subcon-tracted companies that perform cleaning and disinfection services work under a compliance agreement with VS.

Recommendation 7: Develop and implement written operating procedures for APHIS animal import centers to follow that, at a minimum, meet the same standards required of agency approved private quarantine facilities.

APHIS Response: APHIS agrees with this recommendation. VS will review regulations, VS Memoranda, and other guidance documents regarding quarantine facilities for all species, to determine if standards are consistent. If differences in standards are uncovered, VS will then develop a plan (with timelines) for ensuring that operations are consistent at all USDA-monitored quarantine facilities. The review and development of the plan and timelines will be completed by October 1, 2010.

Recommendation 8: Perform bio-security assessment reviews of APHIS' animal import centers to ensure compliance with agency requirements and implement time-phased action plans to correct deficiencies noted during the reviews.

APHIS Response: APHIS agrees with this recommendation and will augment the processes that are already in place for assessing biosecurity. Each animal import center has facility-specific protocols that include cleaning and disinfection procedures. These procedures are evaluated during reviews described in the response to recommendations 3 and 4. VS Area and Regional officials work jointly to correct any deficiencies noted in these reviews. To ensure that current processes are consistent and effective, VS will review all current policies and procedures and will develop a VS Memorandum that addresses biosecurity in the animal import centers and other USDA-approved quarantine facilities. This task will be completed by March 31, 2011, to ensure sufficient time to conduct a complete review and develop clear and consistent policies that can be appropriately implemented.

Recommendation 9: Instruct animal import center directors to enforce all agency policies related to physical security at private bird quarantine facilities.

APHIS Response: APHIS agrees with this recommendation. A VS Memorandum and checklist for the approval of privately owned commercial and other bird quarantine facilities will be developed and implemented by December 2010 to ensure consistent standards for physical security.

Recommendation 10: Require area officials to perform periodic supervisory reviews of biosecurity operations at animal import centers, and provide a method for APHIS officials to verify that reviews are completed and deficiencies are corrected by field staff.

APHIS Response: APHIS agrees with this recommendation and believes we are already in compliance. The station review program, which VS management oversees and is described in VS Memorandum 515.1, includes a review of biosecurity operations and cleaning and disinfection procedures. The reports from these reviews identify deficiencies, if any, and a process is in place to ensure deficiencies are corrected. In this process, the AVIC develops a plan of actions to be taken and sends a copy to the import center, the Regional Office, and VS headquarters. The AVIC is responsible for ensuring that the actions are completed successfully and notifying headquarters when the review is considered closed.

Recommendation 11: Develop a time-phased action plan to implement the recommendations in the 2007 Contagious Equine Metritis report relating to the importation and quarantine of horses.

APHIS Response: APHIS agrees with this recommendation. VS has completed or is working on several actions to address the recommendations in the 2007 contagious equine metritis (CEM) report. Beginning in September 2007, APHIS established CEM coordinators in each state that is approved to receive stallions and mares from CEM-affected countries; the list of state coordinators was updated in June 2010. Training was provided to CEM coordinators in three sessions (April 2008, July 2009, and June 2010).

VS is also in the process of revising its regulations for CEM testing of imported animals. The interim final rule is scheduled to be published by the end of calendar year 2010. Once the rule becomes final, the relevant VS Memoranda will be implemented to update the detailed testing requirements.

VS is developing a database for information (including laboratory results) on imported animals undergoing CEM quarantine and testing. This database is due for completion by March 2011. VS also provided training (in July 2008,

August 2008, and January 2009) to laboratory staff who conduct CEM testing and implemented a process for proficiency testing in November 2009.

Recommendation 12: Revise the user fee rate structure by identifying the funds needed to adequately support quarantine facility operations and upgrades, and at a minimum, update the study for the time it takes to complete all quarantine tasks and establish procedures to periodically update that study to account for time and cost changes.

APHIS Response: APHIS agrees with this recommendation, and has taken the following actions. From July 2009, through January 2010, APHIS undertook a special, internal review of VS User Fees including the animal quarantine facility user fees. The objective of this internal review was to review program costs, estimated volumes, and the user fees structure to identify the properly includable costs. This study will provide information as to where fees should be increased to fully recover program costs, including potential increases in quarantine fees. Phase I of this work is complete.

Subsequent to communication of OIG's preliminary finding, APHIS updated its user fee time surveys for quarantine tasks. APHIS' Financial Management Division (FMD) staff visited the New York Animal Import Center in December 2009, and the Miami Animal Import Center in January 2010, and performed time studies and collected time survey data to use in the next user fee quarantine rate calculations. FMD prepared detailed tables that depict all VS import and export user fees, the dates when time values were updated, and the estimated dates when the remaining fees' time values will be updated. VS has also been conducting internal reviews of costs associated with the quarantine facilities, most notably rent costs.

Additionally, the following actions are planned. APHIS plans to perform an in-depth review of all costs that are recovered through the animal quarantine facility user fees to identify which costs should be included in the fees to adequately support the facility operations and anticipated upgrades. As such, APHIS will include costs identified in this OIG report; costs identified in the APHIS, Policy and Program Development internal review; and additional costs identified by the VS Finance and Strategy Staff. The estimated completion date is August 31, 2010. APHIS plans to complete the update of all VS import and export user fee time values by July 30, 2010. As time values are used to drive costs to various user fee categories, FMD will perform an analysis of how using the updated time values would alter the distribution of costs between various use fee categories. FMD will work closely with VS management and user fee program representatives to develop and propose a new user fee schedule. APHIS will complete the proposed user fee schedule and develop a rulemaking workplan for their implementation by October 29, 2010. Based upon the time requirements for such a rulemaking, APHIS estimates that the new fees will be implemented for fiscal year 2013. Beginning in fiscal year 2011, APHIS will establish accounting codes for individual ports so that port costs can be better tracked. APHIS will also develop periodic evaluation methods to ensure that APHIS has the optimum number of and locations for its port operations.

Thank you for the opportunity comment on this report.

End Notes

[1] Exotic Newcastle Disease is a contagious and fatal viral disease affecting all species of birds and can cause conjunctivitis in people.

[2] These bio-security conditions included single-entry rather than self-closing double doors; torn or inadequate screens over windows and doors; and individuals who were not showering as they entered and exited facilities.

[3] Contagious Equine Metritis is a highly contagious and fast-spreading venereal disease of horses that APHIS considers foreign to the United States.

[4] Animal Health Protection Act, as amended through Public Law 110–246, effective May 22, 2008.

[5] According to APHIS regional officials, there are 16 APHIS-approved private facilities. This total does not include all temporary horse quarantine facilities, such as racetracks, and all State-approved private quarantine facilities for horses imported from countries affected by Contagious Equine Metritis. Contagious Equine Metritis is a highly contagious venereal disease of horses that is foreign to the United States.

[6] APHIS also approves home quarantines, on a temporary basis, for owners of returning U.S. pet birds.

[7] Whether or not a shipment requires a USDA seal depends on the location of the import center in relation to the airport. The Miami import center is located adjacent to the airport and does not require the conveyance to be sealed. The other two animal import centers, at Newburgh, New York, and San Ysidro, California, are approximately 70 and 100 miles away, respectively, from airports and do require an official USDA seal or bonded carrier.

[8] Private bird quarantine facilities may import multiple shipments of birds and quarantine all shipments together.

[9] U.S. Department of Health and Human Services, Centers for Disease Control and Prevention and National Institutes of Health, Biosafety in Microbiological and Biomedical Laboratories, Section IV, Vertebrate Animal Biosafety Level Criteria, Fourth Edition, dated May 1999.

[10] The 131 shipments we reviewed included 89 of the over 1,900 permits (both electronically and manually prepared) and 42 of the over 4,500 release documents prepared by APHIS import staff, and health certificates prepared by foreign governments' veterinarians. A release document is APHIS' approval that allows imported animals to enter the United States.

[11] Exotic Newcastle Disease is a contagious and fatal viral disease affecting all species of birds and can cause conjunctivitis in people.

[12] 9 CFR 93.104 (a) and (b), 93.405 (a).

[13] Not all animals require an APHIS animal import permit, such as certain types of horses (e.g., geldings) from countries not affected by Contagious Equine Metritis.

[14] The total number of shipments is an estimate because APHIS does not require permits for all horse types and some animal shipments may have multiple release destinations. See Scope and Methodology section for statement on data reliability.

[15] Federal regulations do not require a certain language on foreign health certificates, except for commercial and pet birds, but some of APHIS' forms and websites did state that official health certificates must be translated into English.

[16] Country of origin may include an entire country or a region within a country. APHIS has regionalized certain countries that have evidence to show that they can effectively contain an animal disease outbreak.

[17] 9 CFR 93.103 (a)(1)(vi) for birds and 9 CFR 93.304 (a)(2) for horses.

[18] 9 CFR 93.314 (c) and 93.504 (c) allows the import of horses and wild swine from countries affected by Foot and Mouth Disease, but requires special handling and treatment to prevent the spread of that disease.

[19] 9 CFR 93.101 (c)(3) and (f)(3) allows the import of returning United States origin pet and performing birds and poultry from countries affected by Highly Pathogenic Avian Influenza.

[20] 9 CFR 93.302 (c) Cleaning and Disinfection. Whenever, upon inspection, an inspector (port-of-entry official) determines that an aircraft cargo area or shipping container is contaminated with material of animal origin they shall notify the principal operator and cause the cleaning and disinfection under the immediate supervision of, and in the time and manner prescribed by, the inspector.

[21] 9 CFR 93.106 and 93.301 (a) requires quarantine of birds and horses, respectively. 9 CFR 93.314 (c) APHIS allows horses from Foot and Mouth Disease affected countries, even though they can carry the disease in their hooves and on their coat, as long as certain handling requirements are met. 9 CFR 93.301 (c)(2) allows horses from countries affected by Contagious Equine Metritis as long as specific requirements are met.

[22] 9 CFR 93.202 (c) and 93.302 (c).

[23] Animal Health Protection Act, 7 U.S.C. 8301 Section 10404 (b)(1) and (2), dated December 23, 2004, as amended.

[24] 9 CFR 93.302 (c) requires that any conveyance or shipping container that is contaminated must be cleaned and disinfected under the supervision of an APHIS inspector.

[25] APHIS officials informed us that they found one imported horse that may be the cause of the outbreak, but as of July 13, 2010, APHIS had not issued an official report on the source of infection and the cause of the outbreak.

[26] Equine Influenza is similar to Contagious Equine Metritis in that they are both highly contagious and fast-spreading diseases.

[27] The animal import center in California has two locations; one site near the Los Angeles International Airport is used for incoming flights containing imported animals and to escort those shipments to an APHIS-approved private quarantine, (2) the other site is a birds-only quarantine facility located in San Ysidro, California.

[28] The eight privately owned quarantine facilities we visited included six for birds and two for horses. The total number of APHIS-approved private facilities is an estimate because APHIS officials did not maintain a complete list of all private and State-approved quarantines in the United States.

[29] For large commercial shipments of birds, APHIS personnel prepared permits manually. During fiscal year 2008, APHIS issued 99 permits for large commercial bird shipments to be quarantined at an APHIS-approved private facility.

[30] The total number of animals imported does not include semen, embryos, eggs, or fish, which totaled another 45 million animals.

[31] Audit Report 33601-9-Ch, Controls Over Permits to Import Agricultural Products, dated October 2007.

[32] Audit Report 33501-1-Ch, Review of Application Controls for the Import Tracking System, dated March 2005.

In: Live Animal Imports and Disease
Editors: M. Grayson and P. McLain
ISBN: 978-1-62618-275-2

Chapter 3

INVASIVE SPECIES AND E-COMMERCE*

Invasive Species Advisory Committee

ISSUE

Internet commerce (hereafter e-commerce[1]) is a growing and vital part of the U.S. economy. Total e-commerce sales in the U.S. for 2011 totaled $194 billion, an increase of 16% over 2010. From 2002 to 2011, the proportion of reported e-commerce sales in the U.S. grew from about 1.4% to 5.5% of total retail sales (U.S. Census Bureau News 2012). Globally, e-commerce is expected to increase at a rate of 13.5% annually, amounting to $1.4 trillion in yearly sales by 2015 (Enright 2011). A portion of this activity includes the sale and trade of living organisms. Unfortunately, such organisms and other organisms that they may carry can be invasive species, defined by U.S. Executive Order 131121 as "alien [non-native] species whose introduction does or is likely to cause economic or environmental harm or harm to human health." Order 131121 mandates that Federal agencies work to ensure that they do not promote e-commerce in invasive species, because the order states that these agencies should..."not authorize, fund, or carry out actions that are likely to cause or promote the introduction or spread of invasive species...."

A number of government entities have jurisdiction over aspects of e-commerce including particular types of organisms (U.S. Department of

* This is an edited, reformatted and augmented version of an Invasive Species Advisory Committee publication, dated May 24, 2012.

Agriculture, Animal and Plant Health Inspection Service [USDA, APHIS] – plants, livestock and their products; Department of Interior [DOI], U.S. Fish and Wildlife Service [USFWS] – wildlife); shipping services (Department of Homeland Security [DHS], U.S. Postal Service [USPS]); imports and interstate trade (Federal government) and intrastate trade (state governments). However, e-commerce as a sector is evolving and expanding in volume at a rate that may exceed these various capacities to address the associated risks of introduction and spread of invasive species.

ACTION

This briefing paper, adopted by the U.S. Invasive Species Advisory Committee (ISAC), provides:

- Background information on the linkages between invasive species and e-commerce, and
- Recommendations to strengthen action by the Federal government to address the invasive species risks posed by e-commerce.

BACKGROUND

Scientific analyses and informal reviews of commercial websites and specific niche markets in the U.S. reveal a wide range of invasive species for sale, including many species regulated by state and federal laws. Identifying and managing the risks associated with e-commerce is particularly challenging because the Internet simply serves as a mechanism for processing commercial and non-commercial transactions between groups and individuals. Unlike other vectors of introduction of invasive species, e-commerce is not a physical means of moving organisms.

An analysis of the full role of the Internet in the spread of invasive species needs to consider the ranges and amounts of:

- Sectors and species traded: for example, pet and aquarium species, horticultural and agricultural species (plants, cuttings, seeds, soils), live food and bait, scientific and educational supplies, firewood and other biofuel stocks, and herbal or medicinal products;[2]

- Internet tools for the sale or trade of organisms or products that may be pathways for other organisms: commercial websites; auction sites such as eBay; classified ad websites such as Craigslist; online forums such as those hosted by Google Groups, Yahoo Groups, Facebook, Google+, and specialist groups; and other online social networking and communication tools; Actors in supply chains: importers, domestic breeders, resale entities, box stores and large-scale retailers, small businesses, brick and mortar stores, e-tailers, interest groups such as 4H Clubs, collectors and specialist groups interested in particular species, and the general public; and Shipping agents and routes: shippers can include public entities such as the U.S. Postal Service and private companies such as FedEx and DHL; routes of regulatory significance include imports into the U.S. and interstate and intrastate trade.

The scale and diversity of e-commerce present regulatory difficulties. Individuals and companies that sell through e-commerce may not be legally registered businesses and frequently do not disclose their specific location of operation. They frequently fail to acquire the appropriate licenses and permits, or to use appropriate labeling for packages. Sellers that are out of state or out of the country may undermine local efforts with cooperative retailers to limit the sale of invasive species. Sellers can use the relatively high level of anonymity associated with the Internet to skirt accountability and avoid identification, regulation, and prosecution. Shipping agents may not necessarily know they are transporting potentially harmful organisms, or that they are transporting live organisms at all.

A range of scholarly work has addressed various aspects and sectors of e-commerce and other forms of trade in invasive or potentially invasive species. For instance, the Global Invasive Species Program (GISP, no date) provides a broad overview of the issues, Peters *et al.* (2006) examine the horticultural trade in Minnesota, Kay and Hoyle (2001) cover aquatic weeds sold through the Internet and mail, and *Stam et al.* (2006) and Walters *et al.* (2006) focus on the sale of species of *Caulerpa* in Florida. A number of reports have tried to quantify the volume of species being imported into the U.S., including Romagosa (2011) and Defenders of Wildlife (2007) for wildlife, and Smith *et al.* (2008) for fish. Recent studies from other countries include a broad overview of the issues in New Zealand (Derraik and Phillips 2010), an examination of the Internet pet trade in the U.K. (Parrott and Roy 2009), an analysis of the role of e-commerce in the spread of introduced freshwater aquarium fish in Brazil (Barroso de Magalhães and Jacobi 2010), and reports by the International Fund for Animal Welfare (IFAW 2005, 2008) on trade in endangered species and their parts through the Internet.

Live animal imports into the U.S.

From 1999-2009, over 2.8 billion live animals were legally imported into the U.S., the vast majority of which (about 88%) were ornamental fish (Romagosa 2011). Despite the fact that scientific and common names are required and submitted on Form 3-177 or attachments to the form (see Appendix 1), one study found that the USFWS Law Enforcement Management Information System (LEMIS) recorded the full taxonomic data for only 3.8% of all shipments (i.e., those species listed under the Convention on International Trade in Endangered Species) (Smith et al. 2008). Most species also entered without extensive scrutiny of their potential to harm the environment, agriculture, or human health in the U.S. Surveys of aquatic species sold in the Great Lakes region through the Internet and other sources found a significant percentage of known invasive species available for sale, misidentification of species, and high levels of live invertebrates hitchhiking on plants (Keller and Lodge 2007).

A significant portion of this volume in traded organisms can be associated with e-commerce. Experts estimate that there are at least 4,000 businesses and 15,000 individuals advertising reptiles over the Internet. Numbers of e-commercial traders of horticultural species are difficult to estimate, but conservative guesses place them in the tens of thousands (ISAC 2011).

We focus on those invasive and potentially invasive species that are formally regulated by Federal or state governments and thus restricted from trade and transport, such as those listed as noxious weeds or injurious wildlife. Regulation of these species can include prohibiting or otherwise restricting import into the U.S., forbidding movement between states, and prohibiting intrastate trade and other actions controlled by states. In some cases, a species can be regulated, not because it is itself invasive, but because it can carry pests, pathogens, or parasites directly, in packaging, or during conveyance. We divide our analysis into four areas:

1) Issues specific to e-commerce such as composition of the e-retail industry, Internet-related regulations, and on-line vendor and consumer awareness;

2) Relevant issues more broadly associated with commerce such as international and interstate regulations on trade, postal and courier services, species identification, and hitchhikers;
3) Control mechanisms such as web surveillance, outreach and education; and
4) Recommendations to NISC member agencies.

ISSUES SPECIFIC TO E-COMMERCE

The Internet has unquestionably revolutionized how individuals and businesses communicate and make transactions, removing former geographical barriers and obstacles to communication. With regard to the movement and trade of invasive species, three areas are particularly notable: 1) increased diversity of commerce, 2) decreased ability of governmental authorities to implement and enforce regulations, and 3) the increasing role of the Internet in public awareness and education.

Increased diversity: The Internet has vastly expanded the range of people and businesses engaged in the movement and sale of plants and animals. For example, while a combination of large and small "brick and mortar" stores once held sway in the pet and aquarium trade, individual hobbyists, collectors, breeders, wholesalers and others can now easily engage in the sale of species. Some set up Internet-based businesses that cut out middlemen, maintain a low-cost infrastructure, access a broad range of potential buyers, process sales over the Internet, and use postal or express delivery services to send purchased merchandise.

Traditional retailers have likewise diversified by adding Internet and mail sales to their businesses.

This model has expanded the geographic reach of the market, facilitating transactions across the country and around the world.

The array of mechanisms for making transactions is also highly diverse, including standard retail websites, auction sites, local business and want ads, portals that facilitate communication between buyers and sellers, and specialty chat forums and user groups. Social media such as Facebook, Twitter, and Foursquare are further changing the landscape, particularly through informal retail arrangements.

A shift to person-to-person transactions will likely continue, raising significant questions about whether and how e-commerce can be regulated.

Kudzu (Pueraria montana var. lobata)

Pueraria montana (Lour.) Merr. var. lobata (Willd.) Maesen & S. Almeida, introduced to North America from Asia and commonly known as kudzu, is a high-profile, invasive vine. In the southeastern U.S., kudzu is very widespread and forms famously dense blankets over whole trees. Despite this, multiple listings (e.g., "20 Seeds Pueraria lobata Kudzu Seeds") on eBay offer seeds for sale (eBay 2012), and search engines readily find on-line businesses selling seed, such as B & T World Seeds (B & T World Seeds 2012).

Suppliers are motivated in part by Internet sites that host questions such as:

> "Where can I buy Kudzu plants/seeds? Hi Everyone, I would like to buy Kudzu plants/seeds, but everywhere I look, I only see Kudzu destroying products for sale. No plants. I am quite aware of the rapid growth and the capabilities of this invasive species, so please don't tell me why not to buy it. I need it for observation purposes in a closed environment. Thanks, Batman" (Yahoo, no date)

Specialty cultivars of kudzu can also be found on-line:

> "*Pueraria lobata* 'Sherman's Revenge' (Sherman's Revenge Variegated Kudzu) For the gardener who has everything or as the perfect gag gift for a garden party, yes, it's variegated kudzu. Originally discovered in Japan, it was named by plantsman Barry Yinger, who's never met a variegated plant he didn't like. This fast-growing deciduous vine...rumors of several feet per hour when established are probably true...is covered with lovely trifoliate light green leaves edged in white. The vines are adorned with small clusters of Nu-grape soda smelling flowers in late summer. If you're going to have a weed, it might as well be variegated. Not recommended for states where it has been banned, and because there are so many, we won't ship out of state." (Plant Delights Nursery 2012)

Regulations and enforcement: The Internet has facilitated an increase in sales of organisms by individuals, not just by lowering overhead and transaction costs, but also by helping sellers circumvent state and federal regulatory requirements. For example, brick and mortar stores are frequently required by states or countries to apply and pay for licenses that allow them to move and sell species, and for permits to breed or import species into the country. Individuals sellers are often unaware of these requirements or may deliberately circumvent them by being located in another jurisdiction. Such sellers are often hard to trace; it may be difficult to hold them accountable; and efforts by enforcement agencies to pursue them may be time-consuming and expensive.

The Internet has also made it easier to exchange information on how to avoid regulations, such as by falsifying documents or using transshipments, transfers between more than one shipper. Those who want to be responsible may find it hard to find out what the relevant regulations are. There is no one comprehensive listing or guide to federal and state regulations on the transport and sale of plants, animals, and materials that could be a pathway for the transport of invasive species.

Many states lack a standard means for communicating with non-registered businesses that work over the Internet. Policy-makers are still debating whether only in-state sellers should be licensed, how to design the process for licensing, and how to enforce regulations, all difficult issues. Many would argue that current policies have not kept up with the age of the Internet, resulting in an increasingly unregulated sector of trade in invasive and potentially invasive species. The current situation thus favors largely unregulated, virtual sellers, puts conventional stores at a significant competitive disadvantage, and increases the risks of the introduction and spread of invasive species.

Illegal Importation of Freshwater Ornamental Fish

Based on a search of websites, including news articles published on Practical Fishkeeping, there appear to be a number of ways to illegally import prohibited, freshwater, ornamental fish.

One avenue of illegal importation seems to center on websites such as Aquabid.com, where buyers bid on fish offered by a wide variety of sellers worldwide.

As on eBay, fish are sold and shipped to the highest bidder. Some sellers on this website offered fish that were illegal to import into the U.K. and indicated that they would send them to buyers in the U.K. via ground postal service without the import license, health documentation, or notification of the Fish Health Inspectorate required by U.K. law.

In some cases, fish were sent without documentation via EMS Express Mail, a service for documents and merchandise run by postal operators of the Universal Postal Union.

Another apparent route for illegal importation of ornamental fish was for the seller to ship fish to a trans-shipper in a nearby country where the fish were not banned; buyers in the country where the fish were illegal then arranged with the trans-shipper to have the fish delivered to them.

A third means of illegal importation was to falsely declare the contents of a shipment on a custom declaration in the hope of getting the shipment past customs and wildlife inspectors. This may also involve shipping ornamental fish that are prohibited in one country first to a nearby country that does not prohibit them. They are then smuggled into the prohibiting country via ground transport to avoid the more rigorous inspection of international air shipments of live animals.

It is likely that these routes are being used to illegally import prohibited species into the U.S.

Education and public awareness: Perhaps the greatest commercial virtue of the Internet is that it allows individuals to readily find information, albeit sometimes unreliable, about products and sales. Individuals can locate sellers, details of the features and care of species, and information about how to circumvent rules or smuggle banned species. The Internet can also be a powerful tool for educating consumers. A number of targeted efforts in stores and at trade shows, such as *Habitattitude*™ and *Be PlantWise*, have helped educate those involved in conventional, face-to-face transactions. Such efforts are increasing their presence on the web, and there is a need to develop more effective methods to harness the power of the Internet to inform those involved in on-line transactions.

Issues More Broadly Related to Commerce

While the Internet is facilitating a surge in the sale and trade of organisms, it cannot actually serve as a means for the physical movement of species. E-commerce is thus related to a number of other broader areas, including international and interstate commerce, postal and delivery services, taxonomy and species identification, and hitchhikers.

International and interstate commerce: Official federal and state lists of invasive species apply equally to electronic and non-electronic commerce. At the federal level, provisions of the Lacey Act on injurious wildlife allow USFWS to regulate the importation and interstate transport of animal species including wild mammals, wild birds, amphibians, reptiles, fishes, crustaceans, and mollusks that may prove harmful to humans, agriculture, horticulture, forestry, wildlife, or resources for wildlife in the U.S. Importers of wildlife are required to submit USFWS Form 3-177 (Appendix 1: Live Wildlife Import Declarations – Form 3-177). Similarly, the Plant Protection Act of 2000 (PPA) provides for the listing of noxious weeds, broadly defined as any plant or plant product harmful to crops, livestock, poultry, conditions for agriculture, irrigation, navigation, natural resources, public health, or the environment. Under this act, APHIS also regulates the importation and interstate movement of plant pests such as insects and pathogens and the commodities that may carry them. These regulations are named for the sections of the Code of Federal Regulations (CFR) in which they appear. For example, "037" applies to plants for planting and "056" applies to fruits and vegetables. Both the PPA and the Lacey Act work in tandem with the commerce clause of the U.S. Constitution to allow the federal government to regulate trade of potentially harmful species into the U.S. and across state borders.

State governments can similarly regulate the transport, sale, and possession of invasive species within states and many have developed legislation and regulations similar to the Lacey Act and Plant Protection Act that list prohibited species.

Such regulations are also becoming more frequent at the levels of the county and municipality, creating an increasingly complex regulatory system. As noted above, there is no single, regularly updated resource that includes all of this regulatory information and requirements to assist sellers trying to abide by regulations.

Postal and express delivery services: Since the Internet is often used for transactions across significant distances, purchased specimens are generally sent by mail or express delivery services such as those of USPS, DHL, FedEx, and UPS. Such services have their own set of regulations concerning the shipment of species. All packages sent from abroad require a manifest that lists their contents and may be subject to non-intrusive inspection, such as with dogs or X-rays. Manifests for express delivery consignments must be submitted electronically, which allows for advanced targeting through a range of risk screening measures. DHS Customs and Border Protection (CBP) thus has some idea of what to expect prior to delivery of a package sent by express consignment. In contrast, packages send by international mail are currently exempt from the requirement for electronic manifests, which prevents advanced targeting and requires inspection on the spot. Such inspections may or may not occur depending on volume of mail, timing, port of entry, and availability of personnel.

Governmental roles and responsibilities in e-commerce of invasive species		
Agency	Authority	Coverage
USDA/APHIS	Plant Protection Act of 2000: 7 CFR 360 Noxious Weed Regulations	Federally listed noxious weeds
USDA/APHIS	Plant Protection Act of 2000: 7 CFR 319.37 (Q37) Plants for Planting 7 CFR 319.56 (Q56) Fruit and Vegetables	Imported plants, fruits and vegetables that may be invasive or serve as hosts for other invasive pests
USDA/APHIS	Animal Health Protection Act of 2002: 9 CFR 122 Organisms and Vectors 9 CFR 121 Select Agents and Toxins	Animals and animal products that may carry livestock diseases , and permits for moving various pathogens and their vectors
DOI/FWS	Lacey Act: 18 USC 42-43 Importation of Injurious Species (50 CFR 16), 16 USC 3371-3378 Prohibited Acts related to Unlawful Taking of Fish or Wildlife (50 CFR 10-15)	Federally listed injurious wildlife and prohibitions against the import, export, transport, sale, purchase, receipt, or acquisition of fish or wildlife in violation of U.S., state, or foreign law
DHS/CBP	Homeland Security Act of 2002: 6 USC 201-239 Directorate of Border and Transportation Security (7 CFR 319 & 330; 9CFR 94-96)	Border quarantine and inspection stations
DHS/CBP	Homeland Security Act of 2002: 6 USC 201-239 Directorate of Border and Transportation Security (7 CFR 319 & 330; 9 CFR 94-96)	Express delivery services
USPS	Postal Reorganization Act of 1970: 39 CFR 20 International Mail and 39 CFR 111, 121, and 122 Domestic Mail	Postal services
Federal government	U.S. Constitution	Imports and interstate trade
State governments	U.S. Constitution	Intrastate trade

Customs experts have noted cases where multiple shipments of a particularly questionable species were sent under the assumption that at least one would make it through customs and quarantine inspections. Intentional mislabeling of contents can further increase the difficulty in halting the entry of packages containing invasive species.

Shipments of organisms may alternatively travel as cargo, as in the case of some bulk shipments and species relatively tolerant of long times in transit or harsh travel conditions. Shipments are then subject to inspections by CBP and the USFWS. Cargo currently has a significantly lower rate of examination for live organisms than do express consignments or mail. The reasoning appears to be largely that live organisms are more likely to be express shipped than to be transported as cargo in order to keep them viable.

Taxonomy and species identification: Proper naming and identification of species is a major issue in both traditional commerce and e-commerce in live organisms, as for example in the trade in aquarium plants (Thum *et al.* 2011). One problem is that new or little-known species are often particularly sought after. Other challenges include that:

- the exact species may not be known to science;
- the organism may not be identified in the shipment to the level of the species, but rather just to
- the genus, family, or other, higher level;
- species may be incorrectly identified, intentionally or unintentionally;
- a trade or common name may be used that does not refer unambiguously and consistently to
- any one species;
- taxonomic classifications and scientific names can change over time;
- standards for naming and labeling species for shipment and sale do not exist.

Lack of correct taxonomic information obviously makes it very difficult to regulate the import and sale of species, and to assess the volume and risk of trade in a species.

Hitchhikers: In some cases, the major risk may not be from the species being moved, but from "hitchhikers," other species that are moved along with it. Trade in species is a major vector for the introduction and spread of pests, pathogens, parasites, and diseases. Insects and fungal pathogens may be transported on nursery stock, cuttings, growing media, and other associated material. Diseases of humans, livestock, and wildlife health can be carried by introduced fish, insects, and other animals. Packaging, such as soil, water, or seaweed used to pack bait or crustaceans, may include potentially invasive species such as weeds, algae or snails. Solid wood packaging used to transport a variety of goods may be contaminated with insect pests or fungal pathogens. Movement of firewood can present similar risks.

REDUCING THE RISK OF INTRODUCTIONS FROM E-COMMERCE

Despite the breadth and scope of sales of invasive species through e-commerce, there are some positive steps and tools that can be used to mitigate the risks associated with Internet trade in invasive species. Two main types of approaches are through 1) accountability and enforcement, and 2) outreach and education.

Accountability and enforcement: Managerial tools and methods that focus on accountability target the responsibilities of the buyer, the seller, and the intermediaries. Webcrawlers have been used with varying degrees of success to monitor the Internet for the sale of illegal plant materials on a range of commercial sites from eBay and Amazon to Google Groups and Etsy. Enforcement authorities can use Internet tools to identify sellers and to employ a range of responses to address first time and repeat offenders. However, enforcement may need to rely on local personnel to track down sellers and buyers or subpoenas and court orders to obtain electronic transaction data, and those determined to sell harmful species can use aliases, naming practices, and other means to avoid detection. In the case of international vendors, there are few avenues for enforcement at present. Even so, the data collected through these efforts may help analyze trends and assessment of risks, and help those charged with enforcement to better target possible pathways.

Other tools focused on accountability may seek to educate the buyer, for example with on-line warning labels or pop-ups when an invasive species is about to be purchased. This method is often employed by online retailers and catalog sellers, particularly in the nursery industry, and is useful in cases where certain states ban specific species. Requiring electronic manifests with international mail would allow advance targeting of potentially risky packages. Such efforts could be complemented by increased cooperation among DHS, USPS and FWS on border control activities designed to prevent introductions through international mail, express consignments, and cargo shipments. Protocols for consistent identification and labeling could help identify incoming risks and track trade. More generally, adapting existing regulations for postal and express services regarding injurious wildlife and noxious plants to the realities of the age of the Internet and e-commerce would help bring enforcement efforts into the 21st century. There is some concern that better enforcement may drive trade in invasive species underground where it would be even more difficult to track, but little evidence exists for or against this.

Outreach and education: Various mechanisms could be used to increase the awareness of buyers and sellers and their access to information on how to avoid violating regulations or introducing invasive species. A web-based clearinghouse with a constantly updated catalog of federally and state-listed species could be established. Development of resources for scientists to name and for traders to identify species would be useful. Campaigns such as Habitattitude™ that present the problems caused by invasive species could help educate the public. By including general information on the risks and care of species, such campaigns might further benefit trade by educating sellers and buyers about how to maintain or improve the health of purchased species.

Other non-regulatory approaches might include changes in the policies of on-line retailers and commercial forums, informing Internet service providers about the legalities of trade in organisms and their role in respecting them, and developing codes of conduct and best management practices for individual sectors and interest groups. Because codes of conduct or local campaigns designed to discourage use of invasive species could put brick and mortar stores at an economic disadvantage compared to Internet retailers, such campaigns need to work to also influence non-local sales or develop appropriate incentives for local vendors.

RECOMMENDATIONS TO NISC MEMBER AGENCIES

We conclude that relevant federal agencies need to adjust existing regulations and enforcement practices to better mitigate the risks of trade and transport of invasive species through e-commerce. We offer the following recommendations to enhance our collective ability to engage in e-commerce without promoting the introduction or spread of invasive and potentially invasive species.

1) U.S. Fish and Wildlife Service (Department of Interior – DOI) and Animal and Plant Health Inspection Service (U.S. Department of Agriculture – USDA): Expedite listing processes for the national

importation of injurious wildlife and other animals and noxious plants under the Lacey Act, the Plant Protection Act and the Animal Health Protection Act to better assess and address emerging invasive species threats, including those associated with e-commerce.

2) U.S. Fish and Wildlife Service (DOI): Incorporate all species-specific data submitted with Form 3- 177 declarations for wildlife imports into the Law Enforcement Management Information System (LEMIS) or another accessible database.
3) Department of Homeland Security: Expand cooperation with the U.S. Postal Service to monitor and increase the capability to interdict international mail containing potentially invasive species and encourage the U.S. Postal Service to expedite requirements for advance electronic manifests associated with packages sent through international mail similar to current practice for international express mail and consignments.
4) Animal and Plant Health Inspection Service (USDA): Expand the scope of webcrawlers and related enforcement and monitoring activities used by the Smuggling Interdiction and Trade Compliance unit to include a broader array of invasive plants and plant pests, and enhance cooperation with U.S. Fish and Wildlife Service (DOI) to address injurious wildlife.
5) Agricultural Research Service (USDA): Support development of and capacity for an Internet clearinghouse of federal and state-listed invasive species such as injurious wildlife, other animals and noxious weeds and of relevant regulations. Such a resource could be located at the National Agricultural Library's Invasive Species Information Center or another appropriate website and should include relevant agency contact information and a general reporting form that allows the public to report suspected violations.
6) U.S. Fish and Wildlife Service (DOI), Animal and Plant Health Inspection Service (USDA), National Oceanic and Atmospheric Administration (Department of Commerce – DOC) and other relevant agencies: Provide a reference catalog or database of taxonomic resources that commercial interests can use to verify the taxonomic identity of organisms in trade.
7) Department of State and Office of the US Trade Representative: Given that a significant portion of e-commerce entities is based outside the U.S., explore further cooperative and legal measures with foreign trading partners and relevant international institutions and

other bodies to address the illegal import of invasive species into the U.S.

8) U.S. Fish and Wildlife Service (DOI), Animal and Plant Health Inspection Service (USDA), National Oceanic and Atmospheric Administration (DOC): Promote outreach to individuals and businesses involved in the sale and exchange of species over the Internet to reduce intentional and unintentional sales or purchases of species listed as invasive in the U.S. or particular states.

APPENDIX 1: LIVE WILDLIFE IMPORT DECLARATIONS – FORM 3-177[3]

As a general rule, all live wildlife[4] imported into the United States[5] for any purpose must be imported through a "designated port."[6] Under certain limited circumstances, arrangements may be made to use a port other than a designated port. In any event, such shipments must be declared on import and inspected by FWS or a designated alternative, such as CBP.

With limited exceptions, all live wildlife imports must be declared on a FWS Declaration Form, Form 3- 177, as a pre-condition to inspection and clearance before any imported live animals may be released to an importer. Form 3-177 calls for submission of detailed information on the contents of the shipment. The importer must provide, among other information:

- Purpose code (i.e., personal, zoo, commercial, educational, circus, pet)
- Scientific and common names of each species in the shipment
- Quantity of specimens by species in the shipment
- Country of origin
- Transportation code (i.e., mail, air cargo, personal accompanying baggage)
- CITES Permit number, if applicable
- Wildlife source code (i.e., wild, captive bred, ranched)
- Total value in U.S. dollars
- Indication if venomous
- FWS License number if applicable

There are limited exceptions when such declarations are not required. For example, imports of live shellfish and fishery products imported for human or animal consumption, or fish taken for recreational purposes in Canada or México do not require the filing of Form 3-177. However, exceptions are not available if a permit is required under Part 16 (Injurious Wildlife), Part 17 (Endangered species), Part 18 (Marine mammals), Part 21 (Migratory birds), Part 22 (Eagle permits) or Part 23 (CITES). If the shipment is considered a "commercial" shipment[7] of live animals, the importer or exporter may have to obtain an import or export license under 50 CFR Part 14.91.

REFERENCES

B & T World Seeds. 2012. Order item status. (http://b-and-t-world-seeds.com /omasref.asp?sref=2307, accessed March 24, 2012).

Barroso de Magalhães, A.L. and C.M. Jacobi. 2010. E-commerce of freshwater aquarium fishes: Potential disseminator of exotic species in Brazil. *Maringá* 32(3) DOI 10.4025/actascibiolsci.v32i3.3919.

Defenders of Wildlife. 2007. Broken screens: The regulation of live animal imports in the United States. (Washington, D.C.).

Derraik, J.G.B. and S. Phillips. 2010. Online trade poses a threat to biosecurity in New Zealand, *Biological Invasions* (12) DOI 10.1007/s10530-009-9595-0.

eBay. 2012. 20 seeds *Pueraria lobata* kudzu seeds. (http://www.ebay.com/sch/ items/kudzu%20seed?_dmd=1&_sop=12&clk_rvr_id=326663090652 &MT_ID=69&crlp=10758622927_1&tt_encode=raw&geo_id=1&keywor d=kudzu+seed&adgroup _id=2476439767, accessed March 24, 2012).

Enright, A. June 7, 2011. Global e-commerce to reach $1.4 trillion in 2015. *Internet Retailer*. (http://www.internetretailer.com/2011/06/07/global-e-commerce accessed on April 4, 2012).

Global Invasive Species Programme (GISP). No date. The Internet as a pathway for IAS (Cape Town,

South Africa). (http://www.gisp.org/publications/brochures/ FactsheetInternet Pathway.pdf, accessed March 24, 2012).

International Fund for Animal Welfare (IFAW). 2008. Killing with keystrokes: An investigation of the illegal wildlife trade on the world wide web. (Yarmouth Port, MA).

International Fund for Animal Welfare (IFAW). 2005. Caught in the web: Wildlife trade on the Internet. (Yarmouth Port, MA).

Invasive Species Advisory Committee (ISAC). 2011. Special session on invasive species and e-commerce (December 8, 2011, Washington, D.C.)

Kay, S.H. and S.T. Hoyle. 2001. Mail order, the Internet and invasive aquatic weeds. *Journal of Aquatic Plant Management* (39): 88-91.

Keller, R.P. and D.M. Lodge. 2007. Species invasions from commerce in live aquatic organisms: Problems and possible solutions. *BioScience* 57(5) DOI 10.1641/B570509.

Parrott, D. and S. Roy. 2009. A preliminary assessment of a non-native species pathway: The U.K. Internet pet trade (Central Science Laboratory).

Peters, W.L., M. Hockenberry Meyer and N.O. Anderson. 2006. Minnesota horticultural industry on invasive plants. *Euphytica* (148) DOI 10.1007/s10681-006-5942-8.

Plant Delights Nursery. 2012. *Pueraria* (variegated kudzu).(http://www.plantdelights.com/Pueraria/products/308/, accessed March 24, 2012).

Romagosa, C.M. 2011. Patterns of live vertebrate importation into the United States: An analysis of an invasion pathway. Presented at the fall meeting of the Invasive Species Advisory Committee, Invasive Species and Commerce (December 6-8, 2011, Washington, D.C.)

Smith, K.F., M.D. Behrens, L.M. Max and P. Daszak. 2008. U.S. drowning in unidentified fishes: Scope, implications and regulation of live fish import. *Conservation Letters* (1) DOI 10.1111/j.1755- 263X.2008.00014.x.

Stam, W.T., J.L. Olsen, S.F. Zaleski, S.N. Murray, K.R. Brown and L.J. Walters. 2006. A Forensic and phylogenetic survey of *Caulerpa* species (Caulerpales, Chlorophyta) from the Florida coast, local aquarium shops and e-commerce: Establishing a proactive baseline for early detection. *Journal of Phycology*(42) DOI 10.1111/j.1529 8817.2006.0271.x.

Thum, R.A., A.T. Mercer and D.J. Wcisel. 2011. Loopholes in the regulation of invasive species: Genetic identifications identify mislabeling of prohibited aquarium plants. *Biological Invasions* DOI 10.1007/s10530-011-0130-8.

U.S. Census Bureau News. February 16, 2012. Quarterly retail e-commerce sales, 4th quarter 2011. (Washington D.C.). (http://www.census.gov/retail/mrts/www/data/pdf/ec_current.pdf, downloaded on April 4, 2012).

Walters, L.J., K.R. Brown, W.T. Stam and J.L. Olsen. 2006. E-commerce and *Caulerpa*: Unregulated dispersal of invasive species. Frontiers in Ecology and the Environment 4(2): 75-79.

Yahoo. No date. Where can I buy Kudzu plants/seeds? (http://answers.yahoo.com/question/index?qid=20080520220709AAHjrgW,accessed March 24, 2012).

End Notes

[1] E-commerce refers to "the buying and selling of products or services over electronic systems such as the Internet and other computer networks... [and] also includes the entire online process of developing, marketing, selling, delivering, servicing and paying for products and services." While typically associated with the worldwide web, e-commerce can also incorporate technologies such as e-mail, mobile devices, and telephones. http://en. wikipedia.org/wiki/Electroniccommerce (downloaded December 30, 2011).

[2] This list will likely keep growing with the use of new species, end-uses, and pathways.

[3] The regulations contain a variety of exceptions or conditions that apply to wildlife products (dead, preserved, dried, etc.), museum specimens, personal baggage, and household effects, etc.

[4] "Wildlife" includes "any wild animal, whether alive or dead, including without limitation any wild mammal, bird, reptile, amphibian, fish, mollusk, crustacean, arthropod, coelenterate, or other invertebrate, whether or not bred, hatched, or born in captivity, and including any part, product, egg, or offspring thereof." (50 CFR Section 10.12) Domesticated animals (50 CFR Part 14.4) are exempt unless specimens are from a wild population.

[5] Import means any wildlife introduced or brought into or landed on any place under the jurisdiction of the U.S. For imports see 50 CFR Parts 14.61 – 14.62; for exports see 50 CFR Parts 14.63 – 14.64.

[6] There are 18 designated ports, listed in 50 CFR Part 14.12. If special permits are not required, as under ESA or CITES, imports may also be cleared at certain border ports with Canada and Mexico or special ports in Alaska, Puerto Rico, the Virgin Islands, and Guam, provided completed Form 3-177 Declarations are submitted.

[7] "Commercial" means offering for sale or resale, purchase, take barter or transfer for gain or profit. There is a presumption that eight or more specimens constitute commercial use and a declaration is required.

INDEX

C

D

E

F

G

H

I

O

P

Q

R

S

T

U

V

W

Y

Z